# The Really Useful

# ASD

# TRANSITION PACK

# The Really Useful ASD TRANSITION PACK

## Alis Hawkins and Jan Newport

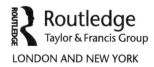

Routledge
Taylor & Francis Group

LONDON AND NEW YORK

First published 2011 by Speechmark Publishing Ltd.

Published 2017 by Routledge
2 Park Square, Milton Park, Abingdon, Oxon OX14 4RN
711 Third Avenue, New York, NY 10017, USA

*Routledge is an imprint of the Taylor & Francis Group, an informa business*

**British Library Cataloguing in Publication Data**

ISBN: 9780863888397 (pbk)

## A word about the authors

**Alis Hawkins** is an independent speech and language therapist based at the mainstream ASD provision where **Jan Newport** is teacher-in-charge.

*The Really Useful ASD Transition Pack* draws on their combined experience of over 25 years' work with young people with an ASD in dozens of schools in Kent.

# Contents

# What is an autism spectrum disorder (ASD)?

We feel we cannot do better than to quote the National Autistic Society. They say:

> Autism is a lifelong developmental disability that affects how a person communicates with, and relates to, other people. It also affects how they make sense of the world around them.
>
> It is a spectrum condition, which means that, while all people with autism share certain difficulties, their condition will affect them in different ways. Some people with autism are able to live relatively independent lives but others may have accompanying learning disabilities and need a lifetime of specialist support. People with autism may also experience over- or under-sensitivity to sounds, touch, tastes, smells, light or colours.
>
> Asperger syndrome is a form of autism. People with Asperger syndrome are often of average or above average intelligence. They have fewer problems with speech but may still have difficulties with understanding and processing language.

People with an ASD can often have accompanying learning disabilities but everyone with the condition shares a difficulty in making sense of the world and the way it is organised.

Asperger syndrome is often described as a form of 'high functioning' ASD. However, these high 'functions' are not evenly spread and it is possible for somebody with Asperger syndrome to be very cognitively able but still experience great difficulties in relating to people socially.

A person with an ASD described the condition as follows:

> People with autism have said that the world, to them, is a mass of people, places and events which they struggle to make sense of, and which can cause them considerable anxiety.
>
> In particular, understanding and relating to other people, and taking part in everyday family and social life may be harder for them. Other people appear to know, intuitively, how to communicate and interact with each other, and some people with autism may wonder why they are 'different'.

The National Autism Society (2011) *What is Autism?* online, www.autism.org.uk/about-autism/autism-and-asperger-syndrome-an-introduction/what-is-autism.aspx (accessed August 2011).

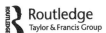

## What are the characteristics of an ASD?

People with an ASD generally experience three main areas of difficulty; these are known as the 'triad of impairments'.

1. **Social interaction** – difficulty with social relationships, for example, appearing aloof and indifferent to other people, or rude and anti-social, or just very awkward in making social overtures

2. **Social communication** – difficulty with verbal and non-verbal communication, for example, not fully understanding the meaning of common gestures, body language, facial expressions or tone of voice

3. **Social imagination** – difficulty in imagining different ways of doing things, different outcomes, and the fact that different minds think different things. This can often cause repetitive behaviour patterns and resistance to change in routine, in addition to a difficulty with 'mindreading', that is, understanding what other people think and feel.

In addition to this triad, people with an ASD often experience differences in their sensory responses – for example, being over- or under-reactive to pain, not being able to cope with bright or fluorescent lights, being hypersensitive to smells, experiencing loud noise as pain, experiencing light touch as painful, and many other sensory responses that neurotypical (non-autistic) individuals find it difficult to understand and sympathise with.

# A few helpful hints

**Parents are not making it up**

Schools often comment that a child seems to demonstrate more radical behaviour and to express more anxiety at home than is presented at school.

A common pattern is for children with an ASD to internalise their anxiety all day at school and then let it out at home, where they feel safe. This may lead school staff to believe wrongly that the child can choose how to behave or that parents are exaggerating, with unfortunate results for the home–school relationship.

**Anxiety rules! (not OK)**

Adults with an ASD often say, 'If you remember nothing else about autism, remember that people with an ASD are always much more anxious than you think.' Worse, this anxiety often centres on things that neurotypical people wouldn't even notice.

Children with an ASD are unlikely to be able to tell you how they are feeling, because they lack either the vocabulary or the self-awareness. This means that the first indication you get that a child is anxious is likely to be some kind of unwanted behaviour.

**Know your child**

No two children with an ASD are the same – what works for one may not work for another.

Like any other child, a pupil with an ASD will welcome the opportunity to build a relationship with you and, although they may not respond to you as warmly as other children do, developing a relationship of trust will make every difference to their school career. You can, literally, be the person who changes that child's life.

Routledge
Taylor & Francis Group

## Please, don't make him socialise

## Is it just bad behaviour?

## He doesn't mean to be rude

**Teacher:** 'Would you like to get on with your work now, Michael?'

**Pupil with an ASD:** 'No thanks.'

The teacher thinks Michael is being rude and sarcastic, whereas Michael thinks he is being polite and answering the question he has been asked. If you think a child with an ASD is being rude, first ask yourself whether they have simply failed to correctly 'read' the question, or the situation – you may just be on different wavelengths.

All behaviour tells us something and 'bad' behaviour in a child with an ASD usually tells us that the child is anxious, stressed or out of their comfort zone. Restoring the child's equilibrium will, nine times out of ten, remove the unwanted behaviour. And sometimes an unexpected behaviour can occur because of simple social misunderstanding. For example, Theo left the room without permission because a small amount of saliva from the teacher's mouth landed on him; he thought he had been spat at and, therefore, was in disgrace, so he left the room.

Playtime is intended for relaxing and letting off steam. But being made to socialise with other children is just not relaxing for many autistic children who may simply want to be by themselves somewhere quiet to get over the stress and anxiety of the classroom. Not having this relaxation may not only impact on subsequent learning but also make socialising in the classroom (eg working in groups) harder, because the child is so stressed that they have no reserves of calm to draw on and no mental space to make use of what they are learning.

## He's OK and then he blows!

ASD brains are not 'wired' in the same way as neurotypical brains. For instance, just to get technical for a second, there are fewer connecting pathways from the limbic system (feeling) to the pre-frontal cortex (reasoning), so children with an ASD cannot use reason to keep the lid on an emotional reaction in the way that neurotypical children do. Emotions can therefore go unchecked and spiral out of control, resulting either in a total withdrawal (eg hiding under a desk, running out of the room) or extreme behaviour (eg throwing something or hitting someone).

## 'What's the time?'

Neurologically, a child with an ASD may have no innate sense of time – the 'clock', which in neurotypical brains lives in a little bit of the brain called the cingulate gyrus, is sometimes simply inactive in the brain of an individual with an ASD. This means that a child with an ASD may spend ages doing something unimportant – such as writing the date – without any sense of time rushing on. In contrast, some children with an ASD become obsessed with the concept of time and will constantly ask the teacher what the time is without actually being able to relate the answer to what is going on around them.

## Sleep

The majority of children with an ASD have significant sleep issues. Some may be able to sleep for only three to four hours a night on a regular basis, resulting in the usual effects of chronic sleep deprivation. Others can't get to sleep until early morning and are always difficult to wake when it's time for school. Some unwanted behaviours may have less to do with 'pure' ASD and more to do with ongoing over-tiredness.

**Humour? What humour?**

Inflexibility of thinking is part of the so-called 'triad of impairments' that defines an ASD. In our experience the more anxious the child is, the more inflexible they become and the less they can deal with change. It is a good idea, therefore, to minimise the number of changes the child experiences because they will find comfort in routine. And because change *will* happen – a burst boiler, an unexpected snowfall – the child needs to be able to rely on a known and trusted adult to help them *manage* the change. It is this adult's job to remain calm (and to keep the child calm) and to show, by the way they respond, that change is OK and not something to get upset about.

**'I'm rubbish! life's rubbish!'**

In our experience children with an ASD tend to remember negative experiences far more readily than they remember positive ones. If 90 per cent of their school day has gone well and 10 per cent has gone badly, it is the 10 per cent they tend to focus on and remember. They can obsess about bad things that have happened to them for months and refer back to these events whenever anything else goes wrong as evidence that life is horrible to them. It might be a good idea to have a 'I have had a fairly good day' sheet to give them to take home. (See page 108.)

**He hates change!**

It is a common belief that people with an ASD have no sense of humour. This is not true. They may not be relaxed enough to show their humour at school but most children with an ASD will respond very positively if you use humour with them because it shows that you are relaxed and comfortable. You may have to explain some jokes to them but it is worth the effort when they start making jokes back. But be warned – to begin with the humour may be very basic!

# Parental Information Sheet

| Name of child: | Person completing form: | Date: |
|---|---|---|

| Situation | Any information you think we should know, eg routines, support given |
|---|---|
| Waking | |
| Dressing | |
| Washing | |
| Breakfast | |
| Teeth cleaning | |

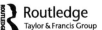

| Situation | Any information you think we should know, eg routines, support given |
|---|---|
| Going to the toilet | |
| Other morning routines | |
| Leaving home | |
| Journey to school | |
| Lunch at home if applicable | |
| Journey from school | |

| Situation | Any information you think we should know, eg routines, support given |
|---|---|
| Arriving home | |
| Eating | |
| Other evening routines if any | |
| Bedtime routine | |
| Sleep patterns | |
| Other adults involved with your child | |

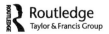

| Situation | Any information you think we should know, eg routines, support given |
|---|---|
| **Siblings** | |
| **Grandparents** | |
| **How does your child deal with callers at the house?** | |
| **Going shopping** | |
| **Visits out** | |
| **Meltdowns** | |

| Situation | Any information you think we should know, eg routines, support given |
|---|---|
| Ways of calming down | |
| Animals or pets | |
| Anything else you think we should know, eg about weekends | |

# Medical Information Sheet

Name of pupil:

Date information given:

Information supplied by: (name)                                    parent/school staff (please circle)

Name of family GP:                          Telephone number of GP:

Is the pupil currently taking any medication? Yes/No (please circle)

If the pupil is taking medication, please give details:

Name(s) of medication(s):                         Medical diagnosis:

1                                                  1

2                                                  2

3                                                  3

Does the pupil have any allergies? Yes/No (please circle)

If the pupil does have allergies, please list them below along with any medication taken for these allergies.
(Please include hayfever.)

Allergy                                         Medication

_____                     _____
_____                     _____

How do these allergies present (eg rash, eye-watering, difficulty breathing)?

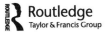

## Medical Information Sheet

Are there any 'early warning signs' that an allergy has been triggered (eg pupil suddenly becoming lethargic or unusually irritable)?

Does the pupil react unusually to illness or injury to themselves? Yes/No (please circle)

If they do, please give examples (eg has meltdown at the sight of own blood, does not tolerate plasters being applied to cuts, thinks they are dying if they have a headache):

Routledge
Taylor & Francis Group
ROUTLEDGE

Has the pupil ever had an operation? Yes/No (please circle)

If they have, what was the operation for and how long did the pupil need to be in hospital?

Has the pupil ever had to be taken to hospital for an injury or for investigations? Yes/No (please circle)

If they have, please give details of the injury or investigations and how long each stay was:

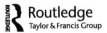

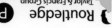

## Medical Information Sheet

Does the pupil have any conditions which mean they have regular visits to hospital or the doctor's surgery for checkups or reviews? Yes/No (please circle)

If they do, please give details of the condition and how often the pupil has to attend hospital or surgery:

Is the pupil receiving any ongoing treatment which means they have to attend hospital, clinic or other venue (eg osteopathic practice) regularly? Yes/No (please circle)

If they do, please give details:

1. Type of treatment

2. Where treatment is given

3. How often the pupil attends

Does the pupil suffer with frequent headaches or other pain? Yes/No (please circle)

If so, what is the preferred method for dealing with this (eg medication, time out, drinking water, calm discussion)?

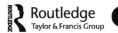

Does the pupil have an unusual response to pain? Yes/No (please circle)

Is the pupil over-sensitive or under-sensitive? (please circle)

If they are, please give relevant examples:

Does the pupil suffer from any phobias? Yes/No (please circle)

If they do, please give details:

Does the pupil have any sensory sensitivities? Yes/No (please circle)

If they do, please give details below:

| | |
|---|---|
| **Hearing** (eg can't tolerate loud noise or specific sounds) | |
| **Vision** (eg bright lights, screens, black print on white paper) | |
| **Smell** (eg doesn't like smells in the environment, will pick things up to smell them, smells people) | |

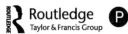

Medical Information Sheet

**Touch**
(eg responds differently to light and firm touch, doesn't like certain textures, can't wear certain clothes)

**Taste and eating**
(eg can't cope with some textures, drinks with a straw, separates food by colour, puts things in mouth inappropriately):

If there is any other medical information not covered on this form, please give details below and continue on the following page if necessary:

Routledge
Taylor & Francis Group

Other relevant medical information (continued):

Signed:

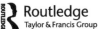

# Why keep a Classroom Record?

Years of working with class teachers have shown us that managing a child who has an ASD is very much a matter of trial and error. Even when you know the child well, you may still not be able to predict how they will react in any given circumstance, and it would not be helpful to suggest that you will. Even parents don't always get it right, as most will freely admit.

So it is a good idea to keep a record of what works and what doesn't with any particular child.

The idea of the Classroom Record came from a newly qualified teacher Alis once worked with (whose name she never knew – sorry!) When she had her first quick 'conference' with him about the child she had come to see, she noticed that he kept referring to a couple of sheets of paper. 'Ever since I started working with this little lad', he told her, 'I've written down the problems we come across and what I did. Then, later, I can look back and remind myself.' He was keeping all the sheets in a folder – purely for his own use – but Alis encouraged him to hold on to them and to pass them on to the child's next class teacher so that they could see the kinds of things the child found problematic and what had or had not worked.

The Classroom Record we have included in this pack is a variant on this teacher's theme. We have added a third box – the one that encourages you to think about what you did when you were put on the spot and to ask yourself whether there was any way you might have handled it better. You may or may not want to fill this one in but it is a way of recording your provision for the child and proof of your ability to reflect on that provision. (We are all being encouraged to reflect on our practice these days.)

Primarily, the Classroom Record is designed to remind you, the class teacher, what you did and whether it worked. We hope it might also be helpful for the teacher who will receive the child into their class at the beginning of the next academic year. They can benefit from a whole year's experience with the child (yours) and, hopefully, not have to reinvent the wheel in terms of strategies and management. It will also provide a useful starting point for discussion with your SENCO if you think the child is going to need more help, or as evidence of your in-class provision when you are reviewing the child's additional needs.

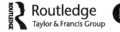

It will also help you fill in the Provision Record (see page 32) as you see whether the accommodations you make on a day-to-day basis begin to form a consistent pattern of provision. Examples are: it becomes clear that the child can't cope with copying from the board because poor attention skills 'lose' the information between looking at the board and refocusing on the book; it turns out that sitting the child next to the window or door or a particular child always causes problems.

We always tell teachers (and parents and the children with an ASD themselves) that knowledge is power. The Classroom Record helps to focus and record that knowledge.

# Classroom Record

| Name: | | Term: | Year: |
|-------|---------|---------------------|-----------------------------|
| **Date** | **Problem** | **Immediate management** | **Ongoing management solutions** |
| | | | |

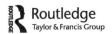

# Classroom Record (filled in)

| Name: Sandy | | Term: Autumn | Year: 2011 |
|---|---|---|---|

| Date | Problem | Immediate management | Ongoing management solutions |
|---|---|---|---|
| 12/9 | Introduced estimates in maths. Sandy finds it difficult to accept the need to estimate answers. Says that he can work out the real answer and that an estimate isn't the real answer. | 'Explained to him that this was part of his Asperger syndrome and exempted him from this homework to avoid a meltdown. | Need to sit down with Sandy and do some really hard sums which he can't immediately work out, so that he can see the value of estimating. Need to make it practical so that he can see the value in his own life and not just in terms of doing lessons at school. |
| 31/9 | Asked whole class to copy title, learning objective (LO) and date from board and then get on with worksheet. By the time most of the class had finished their worksheet, Sandy was still struggling to copy the stuff off the board. | Got Mrs Smith [class TA] to copy from board for him. | Get Sandy to dictate date, title and LO to Mrs Smith so that he is taking responsibility for making sure it's done and not assuming that she will get on with it.\nWhen he can do this, swap over so that he is taking dictation from her – he may find it easier to write than copy. This will help us work out what he's finding difficult, the writing or the copying. |

| Date | Problem | Immediate management | Ongoing management solutions |
|---|---|---|---|
| 6/10 | Introduced fractions. Sandy got very distressed over fractions being expressed in different ways. Said, 'Two quarters is a half so you shouldn't write it as two quarters, it's not right.' | Introduced Sandy to the idea that there is often more than one way to say the same thing. Decimals and fractions express the same reality. A dog can be called a mammal, or an animal, or a Dalmatian – none is wrong, some are just more precise than others. | Need to show Sandy pictures with boxes divided into different reducible fractions, eg box divided into 6. If three are filled in, that is 3/6 – also happens to be a 1/2 but 3/6 is not wrong. Also show him that sometimes it's useful to have things expressed in different ways because it's easier to add 3/6 and 1/6 than a 1/2 and 1/6.<br>Also try to reinforce the idea that things can be expressed in more than one way as he finds this hard in general – always wants there to be only one way to say something ('the right way'). |
| 31/9 | Task was to copy a picture of a Roman soldier from the interactive whiteboard. Sandy said he wasn't going to do it because 'that's Mrs Smith's job'. Mrs S not impressed! | Explained to Sandy that Mrs Smith kindly copies things from the board so that he can get on with the work which goes with the date, title and LO but that in this lesson part of the work was to copy from the board – to learn to copy accurately. He said copying from the board was hard. Agreed that we would print the picture from the internet and he could copy from the picture into his book. | Sandy needs help to distinguish between those times when copying from the board is incidental to the task, and Mrs Smith can be asked if she would mind doing that while he gets on with the real work, and those times when copying is the task and he needs to do it himself. He will need help to work this out but this will be better than simply telling him. |

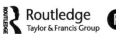

# Why keep a Provision Record?

A provision record does exactly what it says – it records the provision you give to a child from the time they arrive at school to the time they are picked up again.

Why would you want to record things in that level of detail?

As professionals who are currently working in a secondary school, we devised the Provision Record in this pack for primary school colleagues who were concerned about transition from Key Stage 2 to Key Stage 3. They were worried that the level of support that was in place at primary school would not be understood at the receiving secondary school and that the children in their care would struggle as a result. The Provision Record was designed to leave the secondary school in no doubt as to what the child needed and the likely consequences if appropriate provision were not put in place.

But we soon realised that, as any transition can be difficult for a child with an ASD, the Provision Record was almost equally useful from year to year within the primary school. Keeping and passing on a detailed record of provision makes it easy for the receiving teacher to see a quick picture of the child and the support they have been receiving. It avoids the need for long and detailed conferences, gets round the difficulties that arise when teachers leave suddenly without any time for handover, and provides a working document that can be the basis for discussions about management.

In our experience many teachers are not aware of the level of provision they offer the child in their class who has an ASD. 'Oh, I don't really do anything much', they will say. 'I just take it as it comes.' But, when we have taken them through the Provision Record, it often becomes clear (to them as much as to us) that they are offering a very high standard of provision indeed. With the Provision Record (and the Classroom Record that can 'feed in' to it) the expertise built up by a class teacher is not lost when the child graduates to the next year. In fact, expertise can be built on and expanded as the child moves up the school.

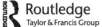

There are other benefits to the Provision Record too:

- It is excellent evidence of good practice for Ofsted.

- It can support and promote good home–school liaison.

- If you have an Individual Education Plan for the child, the Provision Record will show how you are making the plan holistic – not just concentrating on class time but on every minute of the child's day.

- If you are thinking of talking to your SENCO or outside agency about a higher level of support for the child, the Provision Record will show exactly how much support the child requires and – crucially – what happens if they don't get it.

- When you are talking to other professionals (educational psychologists, specialist teachers, speech and language therapists, etc) about the child and their needs, the Provision Record provides a detailed, concise and professional picture of your management.

- It can be a useful planning tool for use with parents when a child with a diagnosed, or suspected, ASD is due to start at the school, whether in the Foundation Stage or as a transfer pupil.

## A quick note about the 'Example' Provision Records

We have included these completed Provision Records so that you can see the kinds of accommodations other schools have made for their pupils on the autism spectrum.

Although Niall, Adrian, Peter, Shona and Steven are not real children, each and every difficulty recorded is taken from working with a real child in a real school. These are the kinds of difficulties that children with an ASD struggle with every day, and the strategies that are recorded here have worked with real children. Unfortunately, that does not necessarily mean they will work with any of your pupils who have an ASD even if the problem seems exactly the same. That's the nature of ASD – it is very, very varied. No two children are the same and even one individual with an ASD can present very differently at different times. Sorry, that is probably not what you want to hear! However, we hope the examples will give you some idea of strategies you might use in your own school.

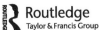

# Provision Record

| Name: | National Curriculum year: | | School year beginning: |
|---|---|---|---|
| **Situation** | **Provision** | | **Reason for provision and potential outcome if not provided** |
| Arrival at school | | | |
| Coming into classroom | | | |
| Seating arrangements | | | |

| Situation | Provision | Reason for provision and potential outcome if it is not provided |
|---|---|---|
| Toileting arrangements | | |
| Assembly | | |
| TA assistance | | |
| Carpet time | | |

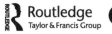

| Situation | Provision | Reason for provision and potential outcome if it is not provided |
|---|---|---|
| **Sensory issues** | | |
| Sound | | |
| Taste and eating | | |
| Touch | | |
| Vision | | |
| Smell | | |

| Situation | Provision | Reason for provision and potential outcome if it is not provided |
|---|---|---|
| Pairing | | |
| Time awareness | | |
| Specialist input | | |
| Small group | | |

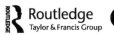

| Situation | Provision | Reason for provision and potential outcome if it is not provided |
|---|---|---|
| 1:1 work | | |
| Break | | |
| 'Who do I go to?' | | |
| Lunchtime | | |

| Situation | Provision | Reason for provision and potential outcome if it is not provided |
|---|---|---|
| Motor difficulties, eg handwriting | | |
| General organisational help | | |
| PE and swimming | | |
| School trips | | |

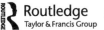

| Situation | Provision | Reason for provision and potential outcome if it is not provided |
|---|---|---|
| Variations, eg art week, book week | | |
| Supply teachers | | |
| Child's area of special interest | | |
| Coping with inappropriate behaviour | | |

Routledge
Taylor & Francis Group

| Situation | Provision | Reason for provision and potential outcome if it is not provided |
|---|---|---|
| Coping with meltdown | | |
| Homework | | |
| Liaison with parents | | |
| Tracking behaviour outside school | | |
| Other | | |

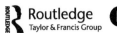

# Provision Record – Niall

| Name: Niall | National Curriculum year: Foundation | School year beginning: 2011 |
| --- | --- | --- |

| Situation | Provision | Reason for provision and potential outcome if it is not provided |
| --- | --- | --- |
| **Arrival at school** | Niall's mum brings him into school early, before the other children arrive, so that he is already engaged in his particular activities when they come into the classroom.<br><br>Miss Singh always greets him and then lets Mr Jack take over as too much language and unfocused social interaction is hard for Niall. | Niall finds it difficult to come into a room full of other children and will not separate from mum in these circumstances, causing both of them distress. Coming into a classroom to be met by Miss Singh (class teacher) and Mr Jack (TA) is calming, especially as Mr Jack can start Niall's 'special games' straight away, making it easier for him to leave mum.<br><br>Niall finds it far easier to speak to adults when he is talking about what he is doing, rather than answering questions such as 'How are you today' or 'Are you ready to have a nice day at school?' |
| **Coming into classroom** | This needs to be carefully managed in terms of what Niall does and what he wears.<br><br>**Clothes and shoes:** Niall is allowed to stay in whatever clothes he arrives in. In wet weather, when this amounts to a very wet raincoat and wellies, this can be a challenge and mum will usually bring a towel to wipe him down so that he doesn't drip everywhere.<br><br>As a move-on strategy, mum is working to find a coat that comes off very easily so that his school clothes aren't disarranged and pulled up (he hates this) when he takes it off. | Niall find the whole process of putting on or taking off shoes and clothes very uncomfortable and distressing.<br><br>To start with, we allowed him to stay in whatever he walked through the door in because otherwise there would be a meltdown and Niall would be unlikely to be able to remain in school. Halfway through the second term (mid-November) we agreed with mum that Niall was probably sufficiently OK with school to begin to break into this pattern because there is always a danger of Niall overheating and his autistic behaviours becoming more pronounced.<br><br>Any change will need to proceed slowly because Niall genuinely finds the process of dressing and undressing physically uncomfortable. Being forced to change can leave him in an agitated and distressed state for the rest of the morning, leading to a much decreased ability to learn and enjoy school. |

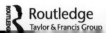

| Situation | Provision | Reason for provision and potential outcome if it is not provided |
|---|---|---|
| **Coming into classroom cont'd** | Similarly with the wellies, mum feels he might be persuaded to take them off if he is allowed to put his slippers on in class because he likes his slippers and finds them comfortable.<br><br>**Toys and activities:** Mr Jack (TA) does turn-taking games and activities to encourage joint attention activities with Niall (as advised by our visiting speech and language therapist) with Brio trains, small balls, bubbles and jack-in-the-boxes. | Niall's mum warned us, before he started school, that he could not share any toy or activity and might hit other children who tried to join in with whatever he was doing. It was decided, from his first day, that we would try and help him to get used to playing alongside others and to develop his ability to attend jointly to an activity in order to build the tools he will need to socialise. An adult is a more suitable play partner than another child as they are able to compensate for Niall's difficulties and 'build bridges' in order to allow him to succeed socially, in however small a way. |
| **Seating arrangements** | Niall is allowed to sit next to Mr Jack when being seated is required (eg storytime) but, most of the time, he is allowed to stand and watch or to wander around the class. He does most of his play activities on the floor.<br><br>Because knowing how to sit down is not a learning objective, we are trying to concentrate on what Niall does instead of where he does it. | Niall has been given a place at a table, like all the other children, but he rarely sits in it as he does not like pencil-and-paper activities and dislikes playing with things such as jigsaws on the table, preferring to sit on the floor with them.<br><br>Being made to sit at the table often results in a fight or in tears and Niall cannot physically be made to stay in his place, which results in disruption for the other children. It is therefore better to concentrate on allowing him to tackle tasks in a way that suits him (and also suits other members of the class, such as Joe who has attention deficit hyperactivity disorder, ADHD). |
| **Toileting arrangements** | Niall needs to be encouraged to go into the toilet cubicle as mum says that the sight of the toilet bowl will usually induce him to urinate.<br><br>Because he has issues with smells (see below) Niall has an intense dislike of the boys' toilets and, instead, is allowed to use the disabled/visitors' toilet next to reception. | If he wasn't reminded by being shown the toilet, Niall would have accidents at least once a day because he has yet to reliably associate the feelings he has in his bladder with the need to urinate.<br><br>The first time he was taken into the boys' toilets he vomited and now flatly refuses to go in. Mum assures us that this is smell related because he cannot deal with strong smells such as the disinfectant used in the boys' toilets. |

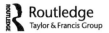

| Situation | Provision | Reason for provision and potential outcome if it is not provided |
|---|---|---|
| **Assembly** | In general, Niall enjoys assembly but he needs to sit next to Mr Jack at the end of a row. He needs to be given something to fiddle with (eg a beanbag or his 'silky cushion') because otherwise he may fiddle with the hair or clothing of the children beside or in front of him, causing them annoyance.<br><br>If puppets are going to be used, Niall needs to be given prior warning so that he can see them and touch them. | Without Mr Jack's supervision, Niall would get up and wander off if he became bored with what was happening or felt like doing something else. Mr Jack can make an on-the-spot decision about whether to try and keep him in assembly or take him out to do something else. Niall is quite capable of arguing for the whole length of assembly (loudly) about whether he should stay or not and how boring it is.<br><br>He is frightened of puppets and human-like dolls, though not of cuddly toys. If he is allowed to look at them beforehand and see that they are just toys and not really alive, he can usually cope, though he needs to be monitored for distress if the puppets are unusually lifelike. |
| **TA assistance** | Mr Jack, the Foundation-stage TA, has been on several courses on the difficulties of children with an ASD and speaks regularly to Niall's mother to ensure that he knows what's going on at home and she knows how Niall has been at school.<br><br>Mr Jack does not spend all his time with Niall even though Niall would like this. | Because of his social difficulties and problems in interacting with the world in ways that other children and adults recognise, Niall needs an interpreter and a champion – not to mention somebody who can monitor his levels of anxiety and try to keep them at a minimum so that he can enjoy school, rather than developing unhelpful strategies just to get himself through stressful situations.<br><br>It is important not to let Niall become over-dependent on Mr Jack because he needs to be encouraged to be as independent as possible, though with support when he really needs it. |
| **Carpet time** | Niall sits at the edge of the group where Mr Jack can monitor him and try to bring him back into focus if he 'wanders off' mentally.<br><br>He is given a fiddling object to keep his hands from stroking other children's hair or fiddling with their clothes. | If Niall were allowed to sit in the middle of the group he would not be able to concentrate on what was being said. Even with prompting he sometimes finds it difficult to listen because he is distracted by other things and – we think – by his own thoughts, but with an adult at his side, there is at least a fighting chance of keeping him listening.<br><br>The fiddling object may help his concentration but it is mainly there to stop Niall annoying other children by touching them. |

| Situation | Provision | Reason for provision and potential outcome if it is not provided |
|---|---|---|
| **Sensory issues** | | |
| Sound | We try to keep the classroom to a low hum anyway, but we know that Niall finds it difficult to concentrate if the noise level goes up and will say that his head hurts. The children know that they are not allowed to shout inside the school building and are encouraged to speak quietly to each other. If there is a loud sudden noise, like clapping or cheering, Mr Jack may need to take Niall out of the class. | If the general classroom noise rises to too high a level Niall becomes distressed and agitated and displays far more unwanted behaviour – for example, hitting other children, shouting, being unable to settle to a task, flapping his hands and jumping up and down. These are obvious signs of distress which rarely occur when the noise level is kept to a working minimum. |
| | We recently discovered that Niall cannot concentrate on anything when the grass is being mown on the school field. He just stands at the window and watches, apparently mesmerised by the sound the mower makes. | We let Niall stand and watch the mower because, at his current level of development, he cannot disengage from this fascinating sound to do other things. However, if he continues to find it fascinating (he may not) we will have to instigate a programme that helps him to tolerate the sound while he does other things. Mum, however, says such fascinations – though intense while they last – rarely continue for more than a couple of months before they are replaced by some other all-consuming interest. |
| Taste and eating | N/A | |
| Touch | Niall is allowed to wear jogging bottoms to school instead of ordinary 'uniform' trousers because they are more comfortable. He is also allowed to keep his outer clothes on in the classroom if he wishes. | Niall is hypersensitive to the comfort or otherwise of his clothes and will complain bitterly if, for example, his mother leaves a maker's label in the back of one of his shirts or sweatshirts, because it irritates him. He likes only what he calls 'soft' clothes, though what is soft or otherwise seems arbitrary to anybody other than Niall, and it is almost impossible to guess what he will and won't like. However, if he is wearing something he calls 'scratchy' he will be fractious and upset all day. |
| | He does PE in his jogging bottoms and school polo shirt to avoid the need to change. | Mum reports that, in order to get him dressed in the morning, she has to let him go to bed naked after his bath, otherwise he will not take his pyjamas off to put his uniform on. |

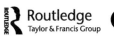

| Situation | Provision | Reason for provision and potential outcome if it is not provided |
|---|---|---|
| Vision | Niall sometimes holds books and other objects very close to his face and will say, 'I'm looking at it carefully'. This seems to be a processing thing rather than a visual thing.<br><br>It's important to make sure that Niall has actually taken in what's on the whole page because he may only be paying attention to very small details instead of looking at 'the big picture'. | If he is encouraged to put items at a normal distance from his face, Niall becomes agitated and protests, 'I can't see it properly! You're stopping me looking at it!'<br><br>Sight tests have shown that Niall's sight is normal, so we think he is 'seeing' things in a different way when he does this, possibly concentrating on tiny details rather than the whole picture. If this persists he may need help, later in his school career, to do it in a less socially abnormal fashion because it marks him out from his classmates in a potentially unhelpful way. |
| Smell | Niall is hypersensitive to smells and often finds them unpleasant. This means that he will sometimes refuse to go into areas where there is a strong smell, for example, the boys toilets. This means that he needs to be given an alternative toileting arrangement. | Niall refuses to use the boys toilets and so has to be provided with an alternative, otherwise his health will suffer or he will have 'accidents'.<br><br>When Niall says that he does not like a particular smell, it needs to be taken seriously. Failure to let him leave the area will result in increasing anxiety leading to behavioural issues and, potentially, vomiting. |
| Pairing | Mr Jack works on paired tasks with Niall and follows advice given by the speech and language therapist to help Niall understand that the person he is working with has a point of view as well. | Niall will work with others on purely physical tasks – eg in PE – but when the task involves making something or some other obvious, visible outcome, he cannot work with a partner because he will always say that the other child is 'spoiling it'. Niall cannot yet see other people's points of view or understand their emotions; he is entirely focused on his own thoughts and feelings.<br><br>This work will be ongoing throughout Niall's school career because of problems with 'theory of mind' – the concept that other people think and feel thoughts and feelings that are not the same as yours – which is poorly developed in children with an ASD, and Niall will benefit from structured input as his brain matures. |

| Situation | Provision | Reason for provision and potential outcome if it is not provided |
|---|---|---|
| Time awareness | Niall has a personalised visual timetable (see page 100) on the table where he sits. This has been made with photos of him taken in school, which Mr Jack and Miss Singh both use with him whenever he asks a question about the time.<br><br>We use a half-hour sand timer with Niall to help him understand the passage of time with reference to his timetable.<br><br><br><br>Mum has bought Niall an inexpensive analogue watch to help him to learn the time. | If left to himself, Niall will ask, several times an hour, 'When is it break time' or 'lunch time' or 'home time?', causing disruption to the class (he will stand next to the teacher until he gets an answer) and upsetting himself because he is unable to feel happy about what's happening next and when it will be.<br><br>On his visual timetable, each section of the day is divided into numbers of half hours (the length of the sand timer) which are 'Velcroed' on to his timetable – three between registration and break, three between break and lunch, etc. Each time the sand timer on his table runs out, Niall takes a Velcro symbol off the timetable and puts it under the flap at the bottom, so that he can see how many more half hours are left before the next thing on his timetable. Though Niall would, initially, spend long periods watching the sand fall through the timer, the novelty of this has now worn off and he only does it occasionally, if he is stressed.<br><br>Niall became obsessed with asking what time it would be 'on the clock' when the sand timer ran out and would stand, looking at the classroom clock. Mr Jack can now answer these questions wherever Niall happens to be, using his own watch, which is less disruptive for the rest of the class and more useful for Niall. |

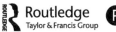

| Situation | Provision | Reason for provision and potential outcome if it is not provided |
|---|---|---|
| **Specialist input** | The local NHS speech and language therapist (SLT) visits six-weekly to advise on programmes set for Niall and to monitor his progress. She is available to be telephoned in the interim for advice on management.<br><br>The SLT has also given the school training in the use of social stories®, which Mr Jack uses with Niall. | Niall is following a programme designed to work on joint attention with an adult (usually Mr Jack, sometimes Miss Singh), using activities that he finds enjoyable. This programme is also running at home with Niall's parents. Without this intervention, he would be far slower to develop the ability to integrate the actions of another person into what he is doing, a skill essential for all types of communication, group work and social activity.<br><br>Without the use of social stories®, Niall finds it very difficult to understand that other people feel and think and react differently from himself and that his behaviour needs to reflect this (ie he cannot just do whatever he likes). Over time, in consultation with the SLT, we aim to move from this approach, which is good for pre-literate children, to the use of comic strip conversations® – using stick men and speech and thought bubbles – to help Niall (and other children) see other people's points of view. |
| **Small group** | When the other children work in a group – usually only in PE at the moment – Niall is carefully supervised by Mr Jack.<br><br>If the other children are able to take Niall's excitability in their stride, then we will try and keep him in the group, but if this seems too disruptive, Mr Jack will choose one or, at most, two other children for Niall to work with. Occasionally, he will work alone with Mr Jack but this is not ideal as Niall wants to interact with the other children. | Niall finds groups of children unpredictable and he is apt to become over-excited and unable to control his own behaviour, for example, flapping, slapping at other children, grabbing at them, or rushing off making noises. |
| **1:1 work** | Mr Jack and Miss Singh work on joint attention activities with Niall daily. | See section on Specialist input. |

| Situation | Provision | Reason for provision and potential outcome if it is not provided |
|---|---|---|
| **Break** | Some days Niall wants to go out and play and others he would rather stay in. If he wants to go out and play the SENCO has organised a circle of friends for Niall and whoever is on playground duty is told which of the friends will be taking Niall to play with them. (This has been organised in class and is shown on Niall's timetable with a photo in a box marked 'My playground friend today'.) Each friend is given a particular game to play – eg hopscotch or skipping or playing on the climbing frame – and the playground duty teacher will keep a watchful eye on proceedings. | If Niall is left to his own devices in the playground he either dominates games so completely that other children don't want to play with him, or will become over-excited and overly physical, charging into other children and sometimes slapping at them. As a consequence, he needs to be guided in his play and to interact with one other child at a time so that he doesn't become confused and 'hyper'. |
|  | If he doesn't want to go out, or if Miss Singh thinks he would be better off doing something quiet, he is allowed to sit in the library and look at the books or play with his Lego while Mr Jack sits and drinks coffee and reads the paper. | If Niall is made to go out in the playground when he is agitated, he doesn't benefit from the social contact but just gets more wound up and stressed so that the next classroom activity is often disrupted. Giving him quiet 'time out' means that he can get back on to an even keel and take part in the next activity more successfully. |
| **'Who do I go to?'** | Niall is not able to monitor his own feelings very well yet and will not be able to say that he needs help when he is upset, distressed or wound up. Therefore, the adults in his environment need to be alert to his mood so that they can intervene if necessary. | It is hoped, as Niall matures and comes to feel more and more relaxed at school, that we will be able to help him become more aware of his own internal state and help him access the appropriate help, whether it's voluntarily taking time out or going to find an appropriate person to help him out of whatever difficulty he is in. This is a long-term goal and will need ongoing input from our SLT. |

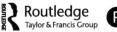

| Situation | Provision | Reason for provision and potential outcome if it is not provided |
|---|---|---|
| **Lunchtime** | Niall has a very restricted diet and brings in a packed lunch every day. Mr Jack sits with Niall while he eats lunch.<br><br>We aim to gradually move Mr Jack away from Niall so that he can sit anywhere at the table, giving Niall more independence and social acceptance. | When eating his lunch, Niall needs to be monitored because, if he sees something in another child's lunchbox that he often has in his own, he may try to take it from them, believing it to be his.<br><br>When Niall first started school, he would not eat at lunchtime unless mum came in and sat with him. This was gradually phased out as Mr Jack sat next to mum, then mum moved to the opposite side of the table, leaving Niall with Mr Jack. Gradually, mum moved from Niall's table to another table, then to just standing inside the door. After Christmas, Niall was able to eat without her coming into school. |
| **Motor difficulties, eg handwriting** | Niall is being encouraged to do pre-writing tasks on the class whiteboard with a thick marker rather than sitting at the table with paper and pencil. Josh and Annabel join him in this, which he enjoys. | Niall dislikes sitting at the table doing pencil and paper tasks. Currently we don't know whether it's the sitting or the pencil or paper he dislikes, but he becomes upset if he's required to do that kind of task, whereas he loves making shapes on the whiteboard. Because it is the motor task we are teaching, not the sitting down, this seems a useful way of allowing Niall (as well as Josh and Annabel) to learn in the best way for him. |
| **General organisational help** | The focus in this area is on encouraging Niall to watch what the other children are doing and to copy them. This means that good role models have to be chosen because he automatically latches on to the most exhibitionist children in the class, not always the most efficient! | Like most children with an ASD, Niall doesn't automatically look to other people to take the lead on what he should be doing. However, this is a major life skill and, if we can encourage him to adopt it now, it will help him in his school career and make him far more independent of adult help.<br><br>It also fits in with the work being done with Niall on joint attention and understanding the thoughts and feelings of others. |

| Situation | Provision | Reason for provision and potential outcome if it is not provided |
|---|---|---|
| **PE and swimming** | Niall is allowed to wear his jogging bottoms and school polo shirt for PE so that he doesn't have to get changed.<br><br>All activities that Niall is engaged in are supervised by Mr Jack or Miss Singh to keep things calm and on track. | As long as he is not made to change, Niall likes PE. He loves running around and the opportunity for physical exercise but sometimes he can 'go over the top' and not stop running or jumping when everybody else does. This needs to be handled sensitively and quietly because any raised voices at this point would only make him more excited and less able to calm down and bring his actions into line with what is required. |
| **School trips** | So far Niall's class has only been on one trip – to the petting zoo. Niall's mum accompanied him on this occasion.<br><br>It is likely that she will need to come on trips for some time to come but, as we always ask for parent volunteers on trips, this does not mark Niall out in any unhelpful way. | Niall finds it hard to understand that the standards of behaviour required at school are also required on school trips. When Niall is excited, fearful or over-stimulated (any of which can happen in a new place) mum reports that he is apt to run off, either to hide or to look at something. As he has no understanding of traffic or stranger danger, this presents an obvious risk to him. |
| **Variations, eg art week, book week** | Niall has enjoyed this kind of variety in the school schedule. He needs to be supervised so that he does not attempt to monopolise new things but, as long as this support is in place, he is fine.<br><br>He needs prior warning if activities are going to include puppets or human-type dolls (see section on Assembly). | Without supervision, Niall behaves as if he is the only child in the room. The need for him to take turns must be explained in advance and his allocated time explained and monitored, for example with a ten-minute sand timer and warnings when his time is almost at an end – 'Only two more minutes, Niall, then it's Sam's go.' |

| Situation | Provision | Reason for provision and potential outcome if it is not provided |
|---|---|---|
| **Supply teachers** | As long as he is allowed to follow his usual routine with his timetable and the usual adjustments are made for him, Niall is not unduly disturbed by changes in personnel. If Mr Jack and Miss Singh were both away (which has never happened yet) we would advise mum to keep him at home. | As long as there is an adult there who can present things to Niall in a way he is familiar with and who is aware of the potential difficulties he might have with particular activities, he is fine. However, if there were no familiar adult present, Niall could easily become anxious and upset, especially if the new adults did not understand his difficulties or the way he usually does things. In these circumstances we would advise mum to keep Niall at home because missing one day of school is preferable to risking a real upset that could have a longer-lasting effect. |
| **Child's area of special interest** | Niall's current focus of interest is colours and he will go around the class naming the colour of every object he can see. He is allowed to do this for specified amounts of time (and quietly!).<br><br>To help him settle to a task, Mr Jack or Miss Singh will sit down with a book of his choice and let him tell them all the colours on a particular page before he starts the next activity. | Niall generally speaks in quite a loud voice and is only now learning to moderate his volume using the 'shh' sign with finger on lips for 'quiet' and 'hands palms down' sign for 'more quietly, please'. This is teaching him to self-monitor and also keeps the class noise level down – ironically, a noisy class makes Niall upset and anxious.<br><br>Sometimes he will not give the book up after this focusing activity, so the adult will leave him to it for a little while until he is ready to engage with the next task. |
| **Coping with inappropriate behaviour** | As long as strategies are in place, most inappropriate behaviour consists of becoming over-physical with the other children. If Niall is supervised adequately, this can be nipped in the bud and his social story re-read to him or the other children's feelings explained calmly.<br><br>It is important to give Niall an alternative to physical contact, for example: 'Niall, instead of hugging Chrissie, you can say, "Hi Chrissie!" – then she'll know you want to be friendly.' | Niall's over-exuberant social advances are meant well but if his physicality is not controlled by the adults around him he will alienate all his peers and end up friendless.<br><br><br>It is also important that he is given help to understand the thoughts and feelings of others and that adults articulate these for him, for example: 'Tom's feeling sad because you bumped into him a bit hard,' 'I'm a bit cross because you did that when I'd asked you not to.' |

| Situation | Provision | Reason for provision and potential outcome if it is not provided |
|---|---|---|
| **Coping with meltdown** | Meltdowns, or uncontrollable behaviour, arise either from Niall not understanding what is required of him – which means that explaining things specifically to him, rather than just to the class, is very important – or from his being asked to stop doing something he is enjoying. When this happens Mr Jack usually takes him out of the class. | If things are explained to Niall he generally copes well with the demands of the classroom, as long as nobody tries to force him to do something he doesn't want to do. <br><br> When Niall 'throws a paddy' over something, it is important not to let this escalate because the more upset he gets, the longer it takes him to calm down. If it looks as if he is going to object to stopping an activity, it is best to take him out of the room – with the toy he is playing with if possible – so that he doesn't distract the rest of the children and upset them. One-to-one, he can usually be persuaded to move on to something else eventually, even if it is something he enjoys just as much rather than what all the other children are doing (this is why it is important to do this outside the class). It is important that Niall is helped to move on from the activity he has become fixated on, even if it is only for one minute, because constantly allowing him to become totally immersed in something of his own choosing will not help develop the flexibility of thought that he needs to live happily. |
| **Homework** | Not applicable yet. However, an approach we feel would work with Niall would be to rebrand homework as 'things we can't do in school because we don't have the right equipment or enough time'. This could encompass finding things out from the computer, picking up objects from the natural world, bringing in cardboard boxes to make things, etc. Once Niall gets used to doing things like this at home, he may be less resistant to the whole concept of doing 'school work' at home. | *[Authors' comment: Many children with an ASD find the whole concept of homework difficult, feeling that school work should be done on school premises, not at home where they relax and do things they enjoy.]* |

| Situation | Provision | Reason for provision and potential outcome if it is not provided |
|---|---|---|
| **Liaison with parents** | When Niall's mum brings him into school she tells Miss Singh what kind of a night he has had and anything else she needs to know.<br><br>At home time, Miss Singh gives mum an outline copy of Niall's visual timetable with one or two words written in each section, for example, 'played Lego® with Jamie', 'skipped in PE', 'did the animal jigsaw' and a smiley, neutral or sad face alongside to show how he felt about the activity. (Niall is being helped to recognise his own emotions and responses to things using these little symbols.) | We are trying to build bridges for Niall between home and school so that he doesn't see them as two entirely different worlds – this is partly to help him develop flexibility of thinking and partly to enable mum and dad to talk to him about school and so encourage and support him. If they didn't have the timetable to tell them what Niall had done, they wouldn't be able to talk to him about his day. |
|  | At the bottom of the timetable, Mr Jack will also write in anything really good about the day that mum needs to know and can help Niall celebrate at home, for example, when Niall was able to take turns in a brief game of throw and catch with another child. | The comments at the bottom of the timetable are key to developing Niall's self-esteem as he – in common with many children with an ASD – tends to focus on what has gone wrong in his day rather than the things that have gone well. |
| **Tracking behaviour outside school** | This is done through daily liaison with mum. | Like many children with an ASD, Niall shows markedly different behaviours at home and at school and we are sharing good practice so that we can adopt the same helpful management strategies. In this way Niall experiences a consistency of approach and doesn't get confused. |
| **Other** | Niall's mum is expecting a baby during the summer holidays and Niall is very confused about what is going to happen.<br><br>This will need careful handling and good liaison between home and school at the beginning of next term. | |

# Provision Record – Adrian

| Name: Adrian | National Curriculum year: 2 | School year beginning: 2011 |
|---|---|---|

| Situation | Provision | Reason for provision and potential outcome if it is not provided |
|---|---|---|
| **Arrival at school** | Mrs Smith (the class TA) meets mum and Adrian and takes Adrian into class while the other children play outside. | Adrian needs a calm start to the day and being in the playground with lots of people coming and going 'winds him up' and makes him agitated. If he came in at the same time as the other children he would be anxious and fidgety instead of calm and ready to begin the day. |
| **Coming into classroom** | Adrian takes his shoes off when he gets in and puts them with his coat.<br><br>Mrs Smith goes through his visual timetable (see page 100) for the day with him, showing him what he's going to be doing and when. Together they put the 'Today' overlay on the name of the correct day of the week and the 'Now' and 'Next' overlays on the correct activities. Mrs Smith asks him when he will need to move them and he tells her. | Adrian has tactile hypersensitivity and finds wearing shoes very uncomfortable. He is allowed to wear trainers for this reason rather than the regulation shoes but still prefers to be barefoot in class. He understands that this means his toes may occasionally get squashed and accepts this.<br><br>Adrian has a very poor understanding of the passage of time and of where he is in the day and week. Without his visual timetable he would constantly ask when things were going to happen, what was going to happen next, etc. A visual reference point helps him to be more independent and means he doesn't have to rely on another person to answer his questions. It also forms the basis of a life skill – using a watch, timetable and diary. |
| **Seating arrangements** | Adrian sits at a single desk at the front of the class and to one side, with his desk against the wall. | Adrian finds it distressing to have other children in close proximity and sharing a desk is an unreasonable and unnecessary stress for him. From his desk he can see the teacher and others but is not distracted or distressed by the other students. He says it 'keeps his body quiet' – if people are close his body gets 'jumpy' and he can't concentrate on anything. |

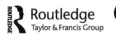

| Situation | Provision | Reason for provision and potential outcome if it is not provided |
|---|---|---|
| **Toileting arrangements** | Adrian is allowed to use the school's disabled toilet. | Adrian is very sensitive about using the toilet and is distressed by the thought of other people coming in and out of the communal toilets while he is in a cubicle. Without use of the disabled facilities he would not use the toilet all day. |
| **Assembly** | Adrian sits with the other children but on a chair, not on the floor. He sits to one side, next to the wall, within easy eye contact of his teacher and the class TA.<br><br>Adrian has earplugs which he inserts before any singing takes place. | Adrian finds sitting unsupported very difficult. He also finds close proximity distressing (see section on Seating arrangements).<br><br>Adrian also finds loud noises (eg singing) very distressing, particularly in a confined space, and his ears hurt. If he were not allowed to wear earplugs he would cover his ears and cry or run out of the hall. |
| **TA assistance** | Some scribing, repeating information that Adrian has not processed, making sure he knows how to begin the task, prompting if he begins to 'wander off' mentally. Current focus in class is on Adrian's problem-solving skills (eg 'What do you think you have to do first?') and on getting him to ask for the right kind of help (eg 'Can you draw these lines for me, please?' rather than simply 'Can you help?'). | Adrian very quickly gets frustrated and discouraged if he cannot immediately see how to do something or do it well. He needs help to begin and end tasks if he is going to succeed and to persevere. Rewards for doing a certain amount of work and for persevering are agreed with Mrs Smith who then helps Adrian achieve these targets, which boosts self-esteem and 'stickability'. Breaking things down into small, achievable steps also helps Adrian succeed more easily, again boosting his self-esteem. |
| **Carpet time** | Adrian is allowed to sit on a chair at the side of the group. | Adrian finds sitting unsupported difficult and would spend his time focusing on his discomfort, not on what was being said. He also has a tendency to fiddle with other children's clothing or hair if he sits on the floor with them, though he does not tolerate being touched himself. Sitting on a chair supports and slightly separates Adrian, so he can concentrate on what's being said. |

| Situation | Provision | Reason for provision and potential outcome if it is not provided |
|---|---|---|
| **Sensory issues** | | |
| Sound | (See also section on Assembly.)<br><br>Adrian finds any loud noise difficult to tolerate and if the teacher is going to raise her voice to the class she warns Adrian that she is going to do this and he puts his hands over his ears. | Without this warning, Adrian would become distressed and be sent into a state of high anxiety. We are also beginning to wonder if he perceives all raised voices as anger directed towards him. |
| Taste and eating | Adrian brings his own lunch and discussion on new foodstuffs (eg when studying healthy eating) is by arrangement with parents.<br><br>Adrian has some food allergies, which are written in his care plan. | Adrian's hypersensitivity to touch extends to oral sensation and he finds some food textures (eg fruit juice or yoghurt with 'bits') difficult to tolerate and may gag. He generally brings his own packed lunch for this reason and should not be made to try new textures without discussion with parents first as his reaction may distress him and/or cause choking. |
| Touch | (See also sections on Assembly and Seating arrangements.)<br><br>Adrian is also allowed to stand at the back of the line when lining up to come into class so that he is not 'sandwiched' between two other children. | Adrian is distressed if asked to stand in line with the other children rather than at the back and will push those on either side of him away, sometimes quite roughly, causing the other children to be wary of him. At the back of the line they welcome him and say that this is his 'special place'. |
| Vision | Adrian is not asked to copy from the board; either he is given a sheet to copy from, or Mrs Smith copies non-essential stuff for him.<br><br>Mrs Smith draws Adrian's attention to various elements on different areas of the page so that he can attend to all of them. | Adrian would spend the whole lesson copying a minute portion of what was required, which would upset him and make it difficult for him to concentrate during subsequent lessons because he would keep returning to his 'failure' in the earlier lesson.<br><br>Adrian does not 'scan' well if asked to look at a whole-page picture or a page of pictures but will home in on detail. Without Mrs Smith's focusing, he would become absorbed in small details and not see 'the whole picture', which would then lead to an inability to complete work satisfactorily or understand the topic properly. |
| Smell | N/A | |

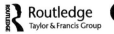

| Situation | Provision | Reason for provision and potential outcome if it is not provided |
|---|---|---|
| **Pairing** | Adrian is allowed to work with Mrs Smith or Mr Temple (class teacher) when paired work is necessary. | Adrian's social skills are not yet at the level where he can see the other child's point of view and, if he is confident of what he needs to do, he tends to dominate the interaction, not allowing the other child a 'look-in'. This would have the effect of alienating the other child or of reducing their self-confidence.<br><br>If he does not think he knows what to do, he will allow the other child to do all the work, contributing very little.<br><br>Mrs Smith and Mr Temple can model good practice and calmly tell Adrian how his behaviour is affecting them. For example: 'When you don't take any notice of what I say, Adrian, it makes me think that you think I'm stupid.' Now that Adrian's reading is at an appropriate level, comic strip conversations® can be introduced to reinforce these comments. |
| **Time awareness** | Mrs Smith is currently working hard to help Adrian to use the visual cues in the classroom – relating his visual timetable to what he's doing 'now' and 'next'. She is also working, along with Adrian's mum, to help him begin to tell the time. They are currently working on 'o'clock' and 'half past'.<br><br>When Adrian becomes 'lost' in time, standing and simply staring or thinking, Mrs Smith gently brings him 'back to earth' by saying, 'Are you away with the fairies again, Adrian?' | Adrian has very little awareness of the passage of time and, without his visual timetable, he would constantly ask Mrs Smith or Mr Temple questions such as 'When is lunchtime?', 'When am I going home?', 'Is it Monday today?', 'Are we going out this afternoon?' Constant reference to his visual timetable anchors Adrian visually in his environment and Mrs Smith now only needs to ask him what we're doing now, and then point to his timetable with the 'today' overlay on, so that he can use it to answer his own questions. This is to help Adrian become more independent and less reliant on the verbal input of others to guide his everyday activities.<br><br>Sometimes, when he asks questions like these, Mr Temple will say, 'I don't know, Adrian, what day do you think it is?' and refer him to his timetable.<br><br>Occasionally, he will say something funny, for example 'Yes, Adrian, we're going to the moon this afternoon!', which Adrian finds funny, if only because Mr Temple laughs!<br><br>When Adrian is 'lost', if he is not brought back to what is going on around him, he can spend minutes at a time concentrating on something totally |

| Situation | Provision | Reason for provision and potential outcome if it is not provided |
|---|---|---|
| Time awareness cont'd | | irrelevant to the lesson but highly relevant to him at that moment (eg the way the sunlight is making patterns as it shines through the fish tank). <br><br> Mrs Smith has explained what 'away with the fairies' means and he finds it amusing, even sometimes saying, 'I'm just going to see the fairies'! |
| Specialist input | An occupational therapy assistant, Mrs Falconer, is working with Adrian once a week to help him form his letters in a more cursive style. | Adrian's handwriting is very effortful and he still finds cursive writing hard. He will frequently say 'I can't do it, it's too hard' and Mrs Falconer is giving him targets to keep him motivated. <br><br> If his handwriting has not significantly improved by the end of Year 3, touch typing will be introduced via a PC game, in order to remove this stressor. |
| Small group | If Adrian is required to work in a small group, Mrs Smith or Mr Temple always sits with the group to facilitate and see fair play. | Apparently daunted by the challenge of having to work with several other children, Adrian will often contribute little or nothing in a group. The mediating adult can make sure that everybody gets a chance to speak. |
| 1:1 work | Mrs Smith takes Adrian through a speech and language therapy 'emotions' programme on a Monday and Mr Temple reinforces it throughout the day, as and when it's relevant, because discussion with the therapist suggests that this will help Adrian more than one-to-one sessions. <br><br> Adrian has two handwriting sessions a week, during assembly, following a programme designed by Mrs Falconer, the OT assistant. <br><br> Mrs Smith does one-to-one troubleshooting work with Adrian as she would with any other child in the class. | Adrian's recognition of emotions – his own and others – is very poor and contributes to misunderstandings and anxiety. If he just did this 'emotions' programme with Mrs Smith, it is unlikely that he would generalise the skills learned into everyday situations. <br><br><br><br><br><br> If Mrs Smith were not available to 'troubleshoot', Adrian would not ask for help but would sit and not complete work. |

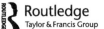

| Situation | Provision | Reason for provision and potential outcome if it is not provided |
|---|---|---|
| **Break** | A 'circle of friends' has been established for Adrian and they will always ask him if he wants to come and play with them at break time.<br><br>If he does not want to play, he is allowed to sit in the office with Mrs Teo (school secretary), reading or drawing, or wrapped in a blanket if he is feeling particularly stressed. | Adrian finds it difficult to join in with play in an acceptable way and needs somebody else to initiate this for him and help him to remember and stick to rules.<br><br>If he is made to go out on to the playground when he wants to stay inside he becomes distressed and will cry or hit out at other children in frustration. Wrapping Adrian in a blanket seems to calm him in a way nothing else does and brings his anxiety level down quite quickly. |
| **'Who do I go to?'** | In the classroom Adrian knows that he can always ask Mr Temple or Mrs Smith for help and that this is always appropriate as long as the adult concerned is not speaking to somebody else, in which case he has to wait quietly until they have finished speaking.<br><br>For break and lunch we have a set of laminated cards showing photos of whoever is on duty and the appropriate one is given to Adrian for him to carry in his pocket to remind him who to go to if there's a problem. His circle of friends also helps him with this. | Because of a lack of flexible thinking and difficulties in forming hierarchies for himself, Adrian becomes very anxious if he does not know who is 'in charge' and whom he should go to if things go wrong or if he needs help or reassurance.<br><br>If he is not told specifically 'This adult is in charge during this lesson, break or lunchtime' Adrian will always go and look for his teacher, whom he thinks of as being in charge of him.<br><br>At break time Adrian is reminded that if any difficulties arise he must speak to the teacher on duty whose laminated photo he has. At lunchtime Adrian finds it hard to speak to any of the midday meal supervisors but he and Mrs Smith are working with Mrs Jellicoe, midday meals supervisor, to try to help Adrian resolve issues with the named person whose photo he is carrying rather than simply to withdraw and come indoors. |
| **Lunchtime** | Adrian finds the noise in the dining hall very distressing, so he is allowed to eat his packed lunch in the classroom where Mr Temple sits with him. | If Adrian were to remain in the dining hall (he is more likely to leave, with his hands over his ears) then he would be in a high state of anxiety and stress during the afternoon and be unable to focus in lessons. He would also be more likely to lash out or shout at other students or teachers because of this stress. |

| Situation | Provision | Reason for provision and potential outcome if it is not provided |
|---|---|---|
| **Motor difficulties, eg handwriting** | Adrian is having help to improve his handwriting (see sections on Specialist input and 1:1 work), but he is also being encouraged to develop basic keyboard and mouse skills.<br><br>Adrian does a variation of the Fizzy programme to help with ball skills (see section on Other). | Without help to improve his handwriting it's unlikely that Adrian will develop legible script.<br><br>Advice we've been given suggests that some children with an ASD never develop fluent handwriting, so we feel it is important to introduce him to keyboard skills even though he is only in Year 2.<br><br>Clearly he needs to be encouraged to persist with handwriting as it is essential in subjects such as maths. |
| **General organisational help** | Adrian uses sequence cards for some activities, for example getting dressed and undressed for PE.<br><br>For tasks such as writing and maths, he uses cue cards and arrows to show him where to start on the page and how to lay things out. Visual organisation aids work really well with Adrian and two or three are stuck to the surface of his desk.<br><br>*[Authors' comment: See 'Some useful practical bits and pieces'].* | Sequencing physical activities is a problem for Adrian and so he may put his clothes on in the wrong order if left to himself, or get stuck 'dithering' as he tries to decide which to put on next. We decided on sequence cards rather than prompts from an adult as the cards provide a greater degree of independence.<br><br>Adrian cannot generalise experience from one day to the next and therefore does not know how the teacher normally wants him to organise his work on the page. He is visually disorganised and has poor right/left awareness and may well start to write at the right-hand side of the page or in the middle, so he needs help with orientation on the page. |

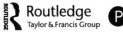

| Situation | Provision | Reason for provision and potential outcome if it is not provided |
|---|---|---|
| **PE and swimming** | Adrian needs close supervision – from either Mr Temple or Mrs Smith during PE. | Adrian enjoys the physical aspects of PE but finds the social side (eg turn taking, remembering when it's his go, remembering what to do) difficult. This will result in boisterous behaviour and/or a meltdown if Adrian is not carefully supervised. |
| | He needs each new activity to be talked through before his turn, no matter how many times he has done the activity before. | Having each activity – whether old or new – talked through calmly and quietly seems to 'ground' him and helps him to focus on what he is supposed to be doing. |
| | Neither adult ever shouts at Adrian unless he is about to do something dangerous. | A raised voice often produces an extreme reaction in Adrian, for example, making him cry and/or run away. However, he responds positively to a calm, measured tone. We try and follow the rule that 'the louder Adrian is, the quieter we get' as matching his tone just winds him up even more. |
| **School trips** | Adrian needs to be provided with as much information about the trip as possible ahead of time. A timetable for the day with approximate timings is essential. If possible, pictures of the place to be visited (eg from previous trips) or of activities to be undertaken are shown to him. | Without this information Adrian has no 'template' for how the day will go and this sense of unpredictability makes him very anxious. He cannot use his experience of previous trips to tell him what this one is likely to be like and needs help to talk this through. |
| | Mr Temple or Mrs Smith always accompanies Adrian's group along with another adult. | Adrian needs to know he has an 'escape route' out of activities he is finding stressful and the knowledge that there is a known adult who will rescue him gives him security and reduces stress. |
| | Adrian should not be allowed to look at a book on a coach journey as this invariably makes him travel sick. | Being sick makes him very upset and he has been known to become hysterical when he cannot have a shower afterwards. |

| Situation | Provision | Reason for provision and potential outcome if it is not provided |
|---|---|---|
| **Variations, eg art week, book week** | The whole school is always prepared well in advance for these events and Adrian is not disturbed by them, often enjoying them more than normal school work.<br><br>If there is a noisy, crowded activity in the hall, Adrian will need to know that he is allowed to go and work somewhere else. | If he cannot leave a noisy environment that he is finding distressing, Adrian quickly becomes upset and will run out of the hall. If he is particularly anxious he may even leave the building and hide somewhere in the grounds. |
| **Supply teachers** | When a supply day is predicted, work is left by Mr Temple who discusses the situation with Adrian and prepares him. In case of unplanned supply cover, Mrs Smith often has to spend a lot of time with Adrian helping him to work or sometimes removing him from the class. | Adrian finds it difficult to cope with change because it is hard for him to generalise from one situation (the class with his usual teacher in it) to another (the class with a strange teacher in it) and transfer behaviour accordingly. To him, a new teacher introduces a whole new ball game, the rules of which he does not know. This often means that he will refuse to do any work and, if not allowed to leave the class, could become distressed and disruptive.<br><br>Managing change successfully is an ongoing goal for Adrian. |
| **Child's area of special interest** | Adrian's current obsession is *Star Wars*. He is not allowed to talk about the films during lessons and, if he introduces the subject, his teacher shows him his timetable and reminds him that the time for talking about *Star Wars* is break time. | Adrian loves to tell you who plays various roles in the *Star Wars* films, to point out that films 4, 5 and 6 were made before 1, 2 and 3, and to quote long extracts from light-sabre battle scenes. If allowed to continue he will also tell you what other films the various actors have been in and what characters they played. Once he begins on one of these monologues he finds it difficult to stop, as if he has started and therefore must finish. So, it is essential to break in and stop him before he gets into his stride, because he will find it easier to drop the topic and focus on his work if he is 'derailed' from *Star Wars* early on. |

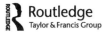

| Situation | Provision | Reason for provision and potential outcome if it is not provided |
|---|---|---|
| **Coping with inappropriate behaviour** | Adrian does not respond well to being told to do things or not to do them simply because those are the rules. He needs to have the reasons for things and the consequences clearly explained. It helps if written and/or graphic material is used (eg comic strip conversations®). | Just being told not to do something is not a sufficient motive to stop Adrian doing something he wants to do – particularly if it is related to *Star Wars* – as the 'push' to feed his obsession is greater than the 'pull' to obey the rules.<br><br>Similarly, if he thinks a rule is 'silly' he will be unlikely to obey it.<br><br>Sanctions are, therefore, occasionally necessary to try and get Adrian to stick to the rules that everybody else obeys. These sanctions usually revolve around not getting a star for that portion of the day to stick on to the photocopy of his timetable that he takes home each evening. As he enjoys sticking these on and his parents make a great deal of how hard he must be working to get all these stars, this does provide some degree of motivation for Adrian. However, a longer-term strategy (explaining why the rules are there and repeating them often) also goes alongside this in the hope that, as he matures, Adrian will begin to regulate his own behaviour without the need for sanctions. |

| Situation | Provision | Reason for provision and potential outcome if it is not provided |
|---|---|---|
| Coping with meltdown | Adrian has two forms of meltdown: curling up under his desk; and losing control and yelling, swearing and throwing things.<br><br>When he 'goes foetal' Mrs Smith offers him time in the quiet area that has been made available for him in what used to be the reading area of the library, behind a set of screens, in a small area with beanbags and cushions. Adrian can curl up here on his own until he feels able to come back to class.<br><br>When Adrian loses control and begins on an outburst, Mr Temple ensures that other children are safe and, as soon as Adrian is able to listen to her, Mrs Smith takes him to the quiet area. Later, when he is calm, she talks him through what happened, using stick man drawings to show events, emotions and consequences. | When Adrian 'goes foetal' he is feeling vulnerable, under threat and very stressed and needs to be somewhere where he can regain his equilibrium. At this point the rational part of his brain is being overwhelmed by the feeling part and until his need for security is met he cannot think or engage rationally. The quicker he has access to the quiet area, the faster he will be able to resume his place in class. If his distress is spotted too late, he may well not come out from under the desk and will need to be allowed to stay there until the next natural break (playtime, lunch or end of the school day) or until he comes out voluntarily. Any attempt to make him come out is counterproductive.<br><br>When Adrian loses control, his anger is in control of him, not he of it. He cannot bring himself under control and think or talk about what has made him angry until his anger has subsided, because the rational part of his brain is – literally – disabled by his emotion. He needs time to let reason reassert itself before the episode can be discussed and what happened can be talked through. Often Adrian does not remember exactly what happened and relies on a reconstruction of the event from an adult's point of view, with stick men drawings, thought bubbles, speech bubbles and a demonstration of cause and effect to help him see the whole sequence of events (the comic strip conversation® approach). |
| Homework | Adrian is happy to read at home, which is his only current homework, but it is likely that, when he enters Key Stage 2, homework will need to be looked at carefully. | Adrian finds school very stressful and arrives home exhausted, wanting only to lie on the settee and watch his *Star Wars* DVDs. Staff will need to consider whether the benefits of his doing homework outweigh the difficulties that Adrian's family is likely to experience in actually persuading him to do it when he is very tired. |

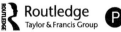

| Situation | Provision | Reason for provision and potential outcome if it is not provided |
|---|---|---|
| **Liaison with parents** | Initially, a home–school book was used but now that Adrian is able to read what is written, he sometimes becomes argumentative about entries that appear critical or negative. So home–school liaison is now done via email with Mr Temple or Mrs Smith emailing home to let parents know what sort of day Adrian has had and any issues that might need clarifying or to be dealt with in some way. | Liaison is essential because Adrian tends to see home and school as two entirely different worlds; getting him to integrate these worlds so that he can transfer skills and strategies is essential. |
| | A timetable for the week with subjects and a rough outline of topics to be covered is also emailed home each week. Each day, Adrian takes home a copy of that day's visual timetable with a star next to each activity that he has completed satisfactorily and a smiley or neutral or sad face to show whether he thought the activity had made him happy, sad or neither happy nor sad. This is so that his parents can engage Adrian in conversation about what he has done at school (informed by the email they have received) and what made him happy and/or sad about the different activities. | In order to strengthen Adrian's episodic memory and his associations between emotion and event, giving him a timetable that he can annotate with his moods and reactions (via the faces) helps his parents to talk things through with him and to 'troubleshoot' events or schoolwork to which he has had a bad reaction. |
| **Tracking behaviour outside school** | Adrian's parents email the school daily to update the class teacher and Mrs Smith on Adrian's behaviour at home and anything he says about school and the work he has been doing, relationships with other pupils, etc. | Adrian's behaviour at home is often very different from the picture presented at school and it is helpful to his parents to know what might have raised his anxiety levels to the stage where he has a meltdown when he gets home. It is also useful for the school to know that Adrian does find his day stressful because this acts as an incentive to us to keep the anxiety down as much as possible so as to make life easier for him and his parents. |

| Situation | Provision | Reason for provision and potential outcome if it is not provided |
|---|---|---|
| Other | Adrian has a special friend – EJ, a Year 6 girl who is a neighbour of his. He is allowed to spend 10 minutes of each lunch hour with her, where she and her friends help him with his Fizzy activities. At the end of this time, EJ takes the ball to the midday meal supervisor and Adrian has to allow her to play with her friends. This needs to be monitored by the midday meal supervisor because otherwise Adrian may pester EJ.

A Social Story™ has been used over the last year to help Adrian understand EJ's feelings as well as his own needs. | EJ, though very fond of Adrian, would become irritated by him if he spent as much time with her as he would like, so she needs to be protected. Adrian thinks that he is EJ's best friend and does not understand why she wishes to spend time with other people rather than being with him exclusively. If his time with her were not monitored and limited, EJ's free time would be monopolised and Adrian would become verbally abusive to her friends. Intervention by the midday meals supervisor would then distress Adrian and make it difficult for him to come into class in a state where he is ready to learn.

Adrian needs ongoing help in learning about friendships because, like all children with an ASD, he is socially immature and does not develop age-appropriate friendships. |

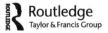

# Provision Record – Peter

| Name: Peter | National Curriculum year: 5 | School year beginning: 2011 |
|---|---|---|

| Situation | Provision | Reason for provision and potential outcome if it is not provided |
|---|---|---|
| Arrival at school | Peter's mum is allowed to bring him into school during the registration period once all the other children are in class. | Peter finds the noise and unpredictable movement of other students coming into the classroom disturbing and it causes him to flap and make a loud noise.<br><br>Next year, when he is in Year 6, decisions will need to be made about whether Peter will cope in a mainstream secondary school with the necessity to move between lessons in crowded corridors full of pushing, shoving teenagers. |
| Coming into classroom | Peter comes in and sits down quietly while the other pupils get on with whatever they are doing. They are used to this routine and make no comment on Peter's arrival. | Peter finds being the centre of attention quite distressing. He cannot interpret why people are watching him and tends to perceive eye gaze as threatening. For this reason no mention is made of his arrival in class and everybody gets on with what they are doing. |
| Seating arrangements | Peter sits at a single desk at the front of the class next to the door. This is out of other children's sightlines as they look at the teacher or whiteboard, so he does not think they are looking at him. | Peter's anxiety levels are very high and he needs to know he can escape easily if things get too much for him. If he is made to sit elsewhere (and therefore cannot see an easy way out) his stress levels become so high that he cannot focus on what the teacher wants him to do. |

| Situation | Provision | Reason for provision and potential outcome if it is not provided |
|---|---|---|
| **Toileting arrangements** | Peter often asks to go to the toilet during lessons. He is allowed to go once during any given lesson and is given a 'toilet pass' at the beginning of the lesson, which he gives to the teacher as he goes out of the class. He knows that if he does not have the card he cannot ask to go again. | Initially, Peter seemed to have some kind of anxiety-related incontinence but he is not incontinent – he just associates feeling anxious with going to the toilet. To reduce the frequency of this behaviour and to help Peter regulate his own anxiety, the card was introduced. Without the card he would ask to go to the toilet several times a lesson and become agitated if not allowed to go each time. The card acts as a very concrete reminder of the rule – one visit to the toilet per lesson. |
| **Assembly** | Peter is allowed to sit with Miss James (his teacher) during assembly and not with the rest of the class. | Peter becomes anxious and potentially distressed in the noisy and crowded atmosphere of assembly and needs to be reassured constantly. |
| **TA assistance** | TA help for Peter is a difficult issue as he does not ask for help and often rejects help from Mrs Branson (the class TA) if it is offered spontaneously. Currently, an approach is being used via individualised worksheets for Peter – next to each written question is a speech bubble which says, 'If you don't know how to answer this question, go and ask Miss James or Mrs Branson'. | Because of Peter's problems with 'mind reading' it doesn't occur to him that other people know the answer to questions that he can't answer. He thinks they must baffle everyone. Having a direct, visual instruction to ask for help if he doesn't know what to do is the most successful strategy to date, though he always goes to the teacher rather than to Mrs Branson for help. |
| **Carpet time** | N/A as Peter is in Y5. However, he would not cope and would have to sit with the teacher. | Peter would not cope with sitting as part of a group like this as the unpredictability of what people might do (eg pushing, shoving or talking to him without warning) would make him very anxious. He would have to sit apart with someone who could reassure him. |

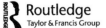

| Situation | Provision | Reason for provision and potential outcome if it is not provided |
|---|---|---|
| **Sensory issues** | | |
| Sound | Miss James gives the class one instruction at a time and waits until everybody has done what she has asked before giving the next instruction. For example, instead of 'Find your history books, write the date, title and learning objective, and then look at the board', she would break this up into:<br><br>• Get your history books.<br><br>• Write the date, title and learning objective like this (putting them on the board).<br><br>• Look at the board.<br><br>If the teacher is giving an extended verbal introduction to a topic, Peter is allowed to read a textbook or a website covering the same material. | Peter has central auditory processing disorder and therefore cannot process speech at the usual rate. He needs the speaker to pause every sentence or two so that his processing mechanism can catch up. He finds conversation difficult for the same reason. Because he can't process questions fast enough to give answers at the usual rate, conversation with him appears stilted. He has been advised to tell people that he has this problem and that it is a common difficulty but he says people will think he's stupid.<br><br>Peter has, independently, found many educational websites that he can access to give him information in a way that he finds manageable and he protests loudly that 'You're not letting me learn' if he is not allowed to access these during the relevant lesson.<br><br>If information is not provided for Peter in visual form he is unlikely to be able to process or remember it.<br><br>Peter cannot follow several minutes of speaking on a topic and does better if given a book, worksheet or website to read covering the same material. If the verbal input has no visual backup the teacher has to go over it again, individually, with Peter.<br><br>Interestingly, we have noticed that this approach has made for far better concentration from the whole class. |
| Taste and eating | See section on Lunchtime. | |
| Touch | The teacher always tells Peter if he is about to be touched (and this is only done if necessary to help him in some way) and will always say, 'I'll touch you so that it doesn't hurt'. | Peter feels light touch as pain though he can tolerate more definite touch (such as being gripped firmly) if he knows it is going to happen. Something like a feather brushing his face would make him scream and flap. Similarly, if somebody brushed past him and a skirt or trousers brushed his bare arm or leg, he would feel that the person had assaulted him. This is a factor in his seating arrangements in class. |

| Situation | Provision | Reason for provision and potential outcome if it is not provided |
|---|---|---|
| Vision | Peter uses a pink overlay for reading black text on white pages.<br><br>He uses a laptop computer rather than a desktop as the screen is less visually disturbing for him (laptop screens don't flicker and, apparently, desktop screens do). | Peter is diagnosed with Irlen syndrome and says that the letters 'wriggle about' without the overlay.<br><br>He uses the laptop very competently and can change the display to colour combinations that suit him. He can, however, become obsessive about changing font colour and size and waste a lot of time in the process.<br><br>*(NB: When applying for statement, need to get provision of laptop written in.)* |
| Smell | N/A | |
| Pairing | When working in pairs is required, Peter works with Mrs Branson or Miss James, using comic strip conversations® to help him integrate their input. | Peter finds it difficult to tolerate another person's input into work he is doing. Comic strip conversations® are used with him in order to help him see that, for social reasons as well as academic ones, it is sometimes necessary to take other people's views into consideration. |
| Time awareness | The emphasis at the moment is on helping Peter to translate 'telling the time' into using the knowledge of what the time is now to guide how much time he has to complete a task. He is asked to work out the time difference between the time now and the time at the end of the lesson and to say how long he has to finish his work. If there are several questions, he then has to work out how long he has to tackle each question. This is being coupled with work on knowing what amount of information it is necessary to give because Peter has a tendency to put down everything he knows. | Peter does not see why he has to do tasks within a certain time and will dash off work that does not interest him in a couple of minutes (or not attempt it at all) and take hours over something that catches his imagination. This will not work in secondary school, so the emphasis at the moment is on helping Peter to pace himself. Currently, Peter is resisting this approach and working to his own agenda! (It does have to be admitted that he is capable of producing work of exceptional quality when allowed free rein, but this will not fit in with how secondary school works.) |
| Specialist input | No specialist teachers are involved with Peter. | |

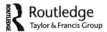

| Situation | Provision | Reason for provision and potential outcome if it is not provided |
|---|---|---|
| **Small group** | Peter finds group work highly stressful and is allowed to work with Mrs Branson or Miss James. (See section on Pairing.) | Peter's auditory processing disorder means he cannot process speech quickly enough to contribute to group discussion and, if required to do so, becomes highly anxious and disorientated, which sometimes leads to a 'foetal curl' meltdown.<br><br>Also, his interaction skills are not yet at the stage where he can see the other person's point of view and integrate it with his own to come to some kind of compromise or consensus. He is still at the stage where he thinks one view must be right and the other point of view, by definition, wrong. This makes productive group work, as the National Curriculum envisages it, impossible. |
| **1:1 work** | Peter is working on a speech and language programme which focuses on interpreting other people's emotions and motivations. He does this work with Mrs Branson but the aims and objectives are carried over into class to help him generalise the skills he is learning. | Peter has great problems 'reading' people's faces and his poorly developed 'theory of mind' means that he interprets other people's actions as if they know and believe everything he does. This means that he finds it very difficult to explain anything coherently because he leaves out important details, thinking that the person he's talking to already knows the whole situation.<br><br>He also assumes that if somebody does something he dislikes, for example laughing loudly near him, they have done it deliberately because they hate him. |
| **Break** | No demands are made on Peter at break time. He is allowed to walk up and down the side of the playground as he prefers to do. Wet play is spent using his laptop with headphones on. | Peter needs to 'tune out' from social demands at break time and his preferred method of 'zoning out' is to walk up and down the side of the playground, with his head down muttering to himself. This seems to calm him and allow him to vent his anxiety. Wet play is more of a difficult time for him because it is hard to get away from other people, but the noise-excluding effects of the headphones and the fact that he is facing away from the others seems a reasonable substitute for his solitary walk. |

| Situation | Provision | Reason for provision and potential outcome if it is not provided |
|---|---|---|
| **'Who do I go to?'** | Peter will not ask for help, so the responsibility for monitoring him during unstructured times falls on the adults in his environment. | Because of his social difficulties, it does not occur to Peter that other people might be able to help if he is in difficulty. To him, it follows that if he doesn't know the answer to a problem, then nobody does. Work is being done with him, using comic strip conversations®, to try and break down this assumption and to teach Peter some theory of mind. |
| **Lunchtime** | As he lives less than 100 metres from school, Peter is allowed to go home for lunch and return during afternoon registration. | Peter benefits a great deal from being allowed out of school during the lunch hour as he de-stresses in a quiet and familiar environment. If forced to stay in school his anxiety would inevitably be far higher in the afternoon. There would also be an issue in getting him to eat because he refuses to eat if anybody is watching him. His mother reports that he always eats meals in his bedroom. |
| **Motor difficulties, eg handwriting** | Peter is allowed to use a laptop for all extended pieces of work as his handwriting is effortful, slow and not always legible. However, he is encouraged to write shorter answers and do work which is not easy on the laptop – eg maths – by hand. | If he were not allowed to work on his laptop, Peter would produce minimal work – eg in English or history – where longer passages of writing are required. He seems to be able to think more easily and express himself more fluently when he does not have the barrier of handwriting to overcome. |
| **General organisational help** | We use task breakdown sheets, mind maps® and writing frames with Peter to help him plan work. | Peter has a tendency to fail to start tasks without a lot of prompting. Because he does not know what the end result is supposed to look like (because he cannot imagine something which does not exist), he needs visual examples or detailed writing frames to help him structure and lay out work. Peter can also 'get lost' in the middle of a task. As we do not want him to become too dependent on external prompting, it is necessary to help Peter learn how to use visual aids for himself, to 'scaffold' activities before he starts. |

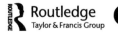

| Situation | Provision | Reason for provision and potential outcome if it is not provided |
|---|---|---|
| **PE and swimming** | Peter does not do PE formally with the other children; instead he is allowed to run around the field so that he gets some exercise. | Peter's gross motor difficulties are such that, combined with his poor social skills, any group-based physical activity is a source of stress for him. (Although he has not been formally diagnosed we suspect Peter has dyspraxia.) An attempt was previously made to follow a Fizzy programme with him but Peter soon refused to do the activities and it became a point of confrontation and was discontinued.<br><br>He enjoys running and swimming, so we encourage him in these activities as a way of keeping him physically healthy and using up some stress adrenalin. |
| **School trips** | Peter rarely goes on school trips. If he does, his mother takes him in the car and meets the rest of the school at the destination. | Peter finds sitting in close proximity to other children on the bus very difficult and would always want a seat to himself. He does not enjoy trips to places like theme parks or other very crowded sites and so only comes on trips to more spacious and less crowded venues. |
| **Variations, eg art week, book week** | Peter is shown photographs of the previous year's activities and talked through what happened. He is then given a timetable for this year's event and walked around the school showing him what will happen in different rooms. Peter always has an exit card which he can use to leave any activity that he is finding difficult to cope with. | If Peter were not well prepared for such a variation in school routine, he would find it extremely difficult to cope with and his high level of anxiety would make a meltdown very likely. If Peter is not allowed to leave activities that are causing him anxiety, he will either run out without permission or go into meltdown. This causes distress and disruption for the whole class as well as having emotional and behavioural repercussions for Peter himself for the rest of the day. |

| Situation | Provision | Reason for provision and potential outcome if it is not provided |
|---|---|---|
| **Supply teachers** | Peter's class has two job-sharing teachers, so each day a photo is put on the board under the heading 'Today's teacher is'. When there is a supply teacher, a digital photo is taken of them and put on the board. The school secretary rings Peter's mother so that she can warn him that a supply teacher is going to take his class that day. | As long as the teacher's photo has been put on the board and Peter has been forewarned he accepts supply teachers without fuss. According to his mother, when told there is a supply teacher coming in, Peter simply asks, 'Will their picture be on the board?' and 'Will Mrs Branson be there?', and if the answers are 'yes' he is content. |
| **Child's area of special interest** | Peter is very interested in astronomy and, as much as possible, we use this as a basis for his other work. For example:<br><br>We couch maths sums in astronomical terms, such as: 'If a spaceship travels at speed x and planet Zog is y miles away from Earth, how long will it take to travel from Earth to Zog?'<br><br>If Peter is required to write in a persuasive style, he might be given the task of persuading some politician to approve, say, a Mars mission. | When his special interest is harnessed like this, Peter will work quite happily and in a focused way which we rarely see when he is not thinking about astronomy.<br><br><br><br>Since the learning objective is about skills and not subject matter, it seems a good idea to get Peter to write about something he is interested in because this has relevance to him. |
| **Coping with inappropriate behaviour** | Peter likes having clearly defined rules and will, on the whole, follow school rules. If he does not, it is because he has not understood the rule or because his anxiety (and consequent need for escape) has overridden his need to conform. | It is *essential* to work out why Peter has behaved in a way that seems inappropriate because he does not often break rules or get into trouble. The root cause of his behaviour will indicate how to prevent him getting into this kind of trouble again. Peter may well not be able to verbalise what happened, how he felt or why he acted as he did, because anxiety 'unhooks' his reasoning skills. Comic strip conversations® may elicit more useful information. Other children may be able to shed light on what has happened but should not be relied on to provide a reasonable explanation of why it has happened, because Peter has, in the past, been used as something of a scapegoat. |

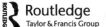

| Situation | Provision | Reason for provision and potential outcome if it is not provided |
|---|---|---|
| **Coping with meltdown** | When he is experiencing a meltdown or is in danger of having one, Peter goes to the quiet room. The class TA will follow him after a minute or two to make sure he is in the quiet room and then leave him for twenty minutes or so, after which she will invite him to come back to class when he's ready. | Peter is a 'runner' who leaves the class and finds a space where he feels safe. Until a special place was provided for him he would hide behind the curtains in the corner of the dining hall. A small quiet room has been made for him out of a store cupboard. It has beanbags, low lighting and a door with a one-way mirror so that Peter can be checked on by staff.<br><br>If Peter had no designated quiet place he would leave school and run home, which involves crossing the road. He would not be able to cross the road safely because during a meltdown he is not thinking about anything apart from getting to somewhere where he feels safe and unthreatened. If he were prevented – physically – from leaving school, he would become more and more desperate and might be a danger to himself or others as he attempted to escape in his distress. |
| **Homework** | Peter is allowed to do all homework on his laptop, with the teacher sending copies of worksheets to his home via email. | Homework has caused a huge amount of stress and family conflict, with Peter firmly maintaining that school work is for school and not for home. He also says he needs to relax at home and that schoolwork 'winds him up'. He loves using his laptop and sees this as recreational and so can be persuaded to complete homework using it. |
| **Liaison with parents** | Peter's mother speaks to Miss James every day after school to see what kind of day he has had, what they have been doing in lessons and anything she needs to prepare Peter for tomorrow. | Peter's parents are trying to break down the barriers in Peter's mind between school and home and try and bring out the common elements, to follow up some of the things he does at school so that he becomes more flexible in where 'work' is done. Having his parents talk about things which are going to happen at school as well as his teachers also helps to integrate the two different parts of Peter's world. Peter has pictures of different parts of the school in a scrapbook at home so that he can show his parents where different activities are done. |

| Situation | Provision | Reason for provision and potential outcome if it is not provided |
|---|---|---|
| **Tracking behaviour outside school** | Peter's mother keeps a log of his behaviour at home and of his sleep patterns because he often arrives at school very tired. | School staff and Peter's parents are trying to correlate any meltdowns he has at home with what has happened at school because he is often not able to tell his parents why he is feeling so anxious or stressed. If any correlation(s) between events at school and Peter's mood at home can be worked out, then the particular stressors can be addressed either with Peter (to help him overcome his negative reactions) or by trying to remove the stressors from his school life where possible. |
| **Other** | Peter's parents have asked the school to modify the language used to Peter to help him integrate thoughts and feelings better, rather than simply talking to the rational part of him all the time. This involves reducing the number of questions asked, trying to balance the statement of concrete facts with the statement of emotional facts (eg 'This makes me feel really excited', 'It makes me feel cross when you do that', 'It's a lovely day today – it makes me feel really happy'), and commenting on what is going on in a kind of 'ongoing narrative' way. | Peter's parents are following an autism intervention programme which is designed to integrate the rational part of the brain with the emotional part so that Peter can think about his feelings and bring emotion to bear on his decision making. It also helps him form much more successful autobiographical memories, something which all individuals on the autism spectrum have problems with.<br><br>Because individuals with an ASD also have problems with 'self-talk' for self-direction and decision making, commentating on what is going on helps Peter to develop his own inner monologue as normally developing children do from about 30 months old. |

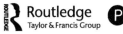

# Provision Record – Shona

| Name: Shona | National Curriculum year: 5 | School year beginning: 2011 |
|---|---|---|

| Situation | Provision | Reason for provision and potential outcome if it is not provided |
|---|---|---|
| **Arrival at school** | Shona arrives at school with the other children and will either try and join in with games in the playground or will stand and watch. | Shona is not really aware of her difference from the other children. Her parents have not shared her recent diagnosis with her as they do not want her to 'play up to the label'.<br><br>Though Shona's attempts to join in with the other children are, at best, clumsy, there is a group of boys in her class whom she identifies as friends and who, while they are not on the autism spectrum, have their own difficulties and challenges. They allow her to join in with their games and will sometimes tolerate her organising them. |
| **Coming into classroom** | Shona comes in with the rest of the children. | Shona's class are quite a rowdy bunch and their class teacher frequently needs to remind them of the rules for lining up and coming into class. This helps Shona because otherwise she has a tendency to boss the rest of the children into sticking to the rules. |
| **Seating arrangements** | Shona sits at a two-seater table at the side of the class, which she shares with Charlie, one of the boys who are her friends.<br><br>She needs to be reminded not to interfere in Charlie's work. | She used to sit in the middle of a run of three tables in the centre aisle of the class. However, she found this uncomfortable as she likes to be able to see anybody who is speaking and would twist around to see a child immediately behind her. As she has little understanding of personal space, this would usually involve encroaching on the desk space of the child either side of her, which irritated them. From her current position, with the wall at her side, she can see everybody in the class without causing difficulties to anybody.<br><br>Her class teacher, Mr Mayhew, has put a small notice on Shona's side of the desk – 'Do your work and let Charlie do his' – which he draws her attention to whenever it looks as if she's trying to help or organise Charlie. |

| Situation | Provision | Reason for provision and potential outcome if it is not provided |
|---|---|---|
| Toileting arrangements | Shona uses the girls' toilets without any problems but the number of times she asks to go needs to be carefully monitored. | Mr Mayhew and Mrs O'Shea have to monitor Shona's level of anxiety because, if she is finding work hard or if she has had an argument with one of her friends, she will ask to go to the toilet and then spend a protracted amount of time there instead of coming back to class.<br><br>If Mr Mayhew sees that she is uneasy or uncomfortable (she squirms about in her chair when this is the case, and winds her hair around one finger) he will usually ask her to come and help him with some task outside the class, eg photocopying, so that he can try and find out what the problem is. Shona will usually tell him without apparent embarrassment – for example, 'Those sums are too hard for me' or 'At break time Luke called me a silly cow and I hit him and now he won't be my friend'. |
| Assembly | Shona is keen to sit with her friends and this is allowed as long as she does not call out too much. | When questions are asked, Shona finds it very difficult, both in class and in assembly, to remember to put her hand up. She will just shout out the answer and, as she tends to speak quite loudly anyway, this is difficult to ignore. Mr Mayhew will take her aside before assembly and remind her that other children need to be given the chance to show that they know the answer as well and that it makes them sad if she always answers first. Shona needs to be reassured that she will be picked to give the answer sometimes. |
| TA assistance | The class TA, Mrs O'Shea, obviously knows Shona's diagnosis and tries, discreetly, to guide her interactions with the other children, particularly the girls, who find Shona 'weird'. She also backs up the need for Shona to allow Charlie to do his own work. | Shona becomes very sensitive if Mrs O'Shea spends too much time with her and will say 'I can do it' or 'I don't need help' or 'Don't tell me what to do all the time' if she feels that her behaviour is being criticised or singled out. This means that any advice and guidance has to be very carefully given and Shona needs to be made aware of other children receiving similar help. |
| Carpet time | N/A in Year 5. | |

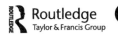

| Situation | Provision | Reason for provision and potential outcome if it is not provided |
|---|---|---|
| **Sensory issues** | | |
| Sound | Shona seems unable to monitor her own volume levels. She speaks in a loud voice the whole time – even her whisper can be heard by the whole class – and she seems unaware of this. | We have requested advice from the schools' speech and language therapy service but, due to 'recruitment issues', there is no therapist covering our school at the moment. |
| Taste and eating | N/A | |
| Touch | N/A | |
| Vision | N/A | |
| Smell | N/A | |
| **Pairing** | Although they are poorly matched in terms of ability, Shona prefers to work with Charlie or Luke, who are her friends.<br><br>Mrs O'Shea and Mr Mayhew will usually take it in turns to hover around the pairing to make sure that Shona's partner doesn't get steamrollered by her rather unsubtle idea of team working. | If Shona is asked to work with one of the more able children in the class, reflecting her own ability, neither she nor the other child is happy. She is apt to be bossy and finds it hard to listen to the other person or include their ideas. Most of the girls flatly refuse to work with her as she is prone to ask intrusive questions – for example, 'Why do you do your hair like that? A pony tail is much more practical for school.' |

| Situation | Provision | Reason for provision and potential outcome if it is not provided |
|---|---|---|
| Time awareness | Shona shows little time awareness and needs constant reminders to finish her work with the rest of the class. She has rejected sand-timers on her desk as nobody else uses one and does not respond well to having 'time checks' built in to worksheets as she gets muddled over reading the clock. Mr Mayhew tries to give general instructions to the class, such as 'All right, Year 5, you need to finish in five minutes', but has to remind Shona individually because otherwise she will say, 'But you didn't tell me I only had five minutes left.' | Shona's parents report that she always behaves 'as if she has all the time in the world' to get things done. She and her siblings all have allocated chores but Shona always needs chivvying to complete hers as she will take ages doing one small part of what she is supposed to be doing, having forgotten that she still has the rest to do. For example, she will spend a long time measuring out the rabbit's food, trying to equalise the number of green and brown 'nuts' that go into his bowl, forgetting that she has to clean out his hutch and move his run as well. Mum sets a kitchen timer for two minutes, after which Shona has to stop measuring out food and move on to the next task, but Shona will not use the timer in school. |
| Specialist input | Since her diagnosis, Shona is under the care of a paediatrician, but there is no liaison with school beyond update reports.<br><br>We have requested speech and language therapy advice and are awaiting the appointment of a new therapist for our group of schools. | |
| Small group | An adult, either Mr Mayhew or Mrs O'Shea, will always work with any group Shona is involved with. | Without adult supervision, Shona takes control of the group and becomes overly dominant. Only her ideas can be considered and only she is allowed to do the practical, hands-on elements. In her mind, she knows how to do everything and just needs to be allowed to get on with it. The adult present can emphasise her good ideas but can also quietly point out to her what effect her behaviour is having on the rest of the group.<br><br>After the first group-based activity in Year 5 was less than successful (not just in Shona's group) Mr Mayhew got the class to come up with their own rules for group work, which include things such as listening to everybody's opinion, not saying anything negative. These rules are read at the beginning of each group work activity and this benefits Shona greatly. They are also printed and put on each table so that they can be referred to if behaviour begins to slip. |

| Situation | Provision | Reason for provision and potential outcome if it is not provided |
|---|---|---|
| **1:1 work** | The whole school is currently following a programme to develop the pupils' emotional intelligence and Shona has extra sessions with Mrs O'Shea on some of these activities. | A number of the children in the class go out for extra tuition of one kind or another – reading, maths, etc – so Shona does not feel singled out in having this extra session.<br><br>The sessions work on discussing cartoon pictures of situations and the emotions each person is likely to be feeling and why. These emotions are then related to situations Shona has encountered in school in order to generalise the learning to her own circumstance. |
| **Break** | Shona usually manages to play without too much incident with Charlie and Luke and their friends but, if the adult on duty spots her getting into difficulties, they will find a job for her to do and talk to her later about what was happening. | Shona is not good at repairing situations once they have begun to break down and little niggles often result in a huge shouting match and her flouncing off or hitting one of the boys. This leaves her angry and hurt and unable to settle for the rest of the day. She will mutter to herself and send threatening looks at her new 'enemy', which is unsettling for other children as well.<br><br>She is usually unable to say what has gone wrong and will always attribute blame to somebody else rather than seeing her own part in the conflict. This is one of the things that the emotional intelligence sessions are trying to address. |

| Situation | Provision | Reason for provision and potential outcome if it is not provided |
|---|---|---|
| 'Who do I go to?' | Shona does not like asking for help but she knows that the adult on duty at break and lunchtime should be her first port of call if she is in difficulties. | Shona's reluctance to ask for help means that the adult on duty has to be very aware of her interactions with the boys she plays with so that minor spats do not escalate into something more serious.<br><br>Some work is being done with Years 5 and 6 on conflict resolution because a lot of the pupils – particularly boys – would rather resort to pushing and shoving and hitting than sorting things out verbally. Shona needs to have the strategies discussed in these sessions reinforced for her fairly frequently and modelled or demonstrated. |
|  | Shona gets very upset when she sees other children breaking school rules and is encouraged to tell her teacher or teaching assistant rather than confronting the child about it herself. | If she were not given permission to tell the teacher when she sees breaches of the rules Shona would try and sort out the situation herself, telling the child off and trying to give out sanctions. This would, obviously, make her even less popular among her peers than she is already. Mr Mayhew and Mrs O'Shea have an ongoing policy of explaining to her that breaking the school rules, though not a good thing, does not make the child concerned a bad person or a criminal. |
| Lunchtime | Shona's family is vegetarian and she brings in a packed lunch. She sits on a table with the other children who eat a packed lunch, with her back to the children eating school dinners, as she is apt to describe school dinners as 'disgusting' if they contain meat. | Shona's reaction to meat eating has meant that we have had to organise separate tables for those who eat packed lunches and those who eat school dinners so that she is not confronted with anybody eating meat (Shona has been asked not to interrogate the other children about what they have in their sandwiches). This is not about trying not to offend Shona, but is to stop her engaging in arguments with non-vegetarians and to stop her saying in a loud voice, 'Eating meat is disgusting and cruel'. |

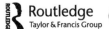

| Situation | Provision | Reason for provision and potential outcome if it is not provided |
|---|---|---|
| **Motor difficulties, eg handwriting** | Shona has good handwriting and writes at a reasonable speed.<br><br>She does not seem to have particular motor difficulties, though she did follow the Fizzy programme (an exercise programme to develop fine and gross motor skills) for co-ordination when she was in the lower school. | |
| **General organisational help** | The whole class is encouraged to use mind maps® to organise and record longer pieces of work and Shona uses this technique well, though she can become distracted by using all the colours in her felt-tip set. | Shona is an able child whose general knowledge is sometimes surprising and who takes in information in the class with relative ease. However, she cannot always produce work of a quality that reflects her ability because of her organisational difficulties, so mind maps® and other planning devices – eg writing frames – really help to structure her work and allow her to show what she knows. She has become something of an evangelist for mind maps® and will help other children to create one if they seem to be struggling. |
| **PE and swimming** | One of the other girls in the class is chosen each lesson to be her PE buddy and Shona has to match her rate of changing to that of her buddy, with the buddy reminding her if she slows down. | Shona needs to be helped when changing for PE as otherwise she could spend the whole lesson folding and refolding the clothes she has taken off because of her inability to see how time is going on.<br><br>The buddy is necessary for the whole of the lesson because otherwise Shona would never have a partner to work with. The other girls do not like working with Shona but, because they each take it in turns to be her buddy, this does not cause too much difficulty. |

| Situation | Provision | Reason for provision and potential outcome if it is not provided |
|---|---|---|
| School trips | Mr Mayhew always makes sure that Shona is in his group on any school trips rather than in a group with Mrs O'Shea or a parent volunteer.<br><br>A very clear timetable needs to be drawn up for the day so that Shona knows what is going to happen and when. | Shona enjoys trips but is apt to become over-excited and to try and take over any group she is in and tell the other children what to do. When she is in this state, only Mr Mayhew can persuade her that she does not need to be in charge.<br><br>Without a timetable, Shona will interrupt activities by frequently asking when they are going to the shops. She is always desperate to spend the money her parents have given her and finds it difficult to concentrate on anything else if she doesn't know when the shop visit will be coming up. |
| Variations, eg art week, book week | As long as the usual precautions are taken to stop Shona taking over groups or dominating any interaction – eg monopolising a visiting adult – these are not a problem. | If she were allowed to, Shona would sit herself in front of a visitor, firing questions at them and engaging them in conversation about similar things the class has done before.<br><br>Mrs O'Shea or Mr Mayhew will usually sit down with her and talk through the visit and emphasise the need for other pupils to have the opportunity to talk to visitors as much as her. |
| Supply teachers | Supply teachers are given a pen-portrait of Shona and her particular needs so that conflicts and misunderstandings are less likely to happen. Mrs O'Shea is available to give advice and this Provision Record is given to the teacher. | Without information from the pen-portrait an adult unfamiliar with Shona would be likely to treat her as a naughty, attention-seeking child instead of one who has an ASD. They might also pair her inappropriately or misunderstand her need to tell them that somebody had done something against the rules. |

83

| Situation | Provision | Reason for provision and potential outcome if it is not provided |
|---|---|---|
| **Child's area of special interest** | Shona knows a surprising number of facts about rabbits in captivity.<br><br>She is allowed to mention one fact about rabbits in class if it is relevant to the discussion but not otherwise. This is part of an ongoing effort to get Shona to try and match what she says to what is being discussed because she will often go off at a tangent on to thoughts that have been sparked off by the subject under discussion. | Shona is prone to talk at length about her pet rabbits and will do so at the slightest opportunity. She has photographs of them and video clips on her mobile phone.<br><br>Without rules about how often she is allowed to mention her rabbits – or rabbits in general – Shona would talk about them incessantly and would hold up lessons in doing so.<br><br>Discussions will often lead to her making comments that are not specifically relevant to what we are working on, which shows that her understanding is sometimes confused by the tendency of her thought processes to go off at tangents. This means that it is essential to bring her gently but firmly back on to the real subject under discussion, to make sure she is following what is going on; otherwise, her recollection of the lesson may be cluttered up with a whole raft of irrelevant associations that her brain has made. |
| **Coping with inappropriate behaviour** | There has been whole-school discussion at staff meetings about a consistent approach to Shona's behaviours, particularly her policing of other children and bossiness towards them. It has been agreed and acknowledged that, however irritating her behaviour may be to adults, it is beyond her control at the moment and is a part of her ASD which needs focused work and help. | It would be easy to be irritated by Shona's behaviour and rather 'in your face' style if the reason for it were not clear and reinforced regularly. As she is dependent on the adults around her to help her to regulate her interactions with her peers, Shona needs staff to be sympathetic to her needs and keen to help her to be a more successful communicator. |
| **Coping with meltdown** | Shona has never had a meltdown at school, though her parents say she does occasionally shout and scream and end up in a crying fit at home.<br><br>They have asked that, if she ever does lose control at school, they should be called so that they can come and fetch her. | |

Routledge
Taylor & Francis Group

| Situation | Provision | Reason for provision and potential outcome if it is not provided |
|---|---|---|
| Homework | Shona's homework is written down for her by Mr Mayhew, along with the time that should be spent on it. | Shona is prone to misremember what she has to do and, when her parents try to help sort things out, loses her temper with them. When her homework is written down, the task is clear and she is happier for her parents to help as she is more confident that both they and she know what is being asked. The time recommendation is necessary as otherwise Shona might spend two hours on a piece of internet research that should take ten minutes. |
| Liaison with parents | We have regular monthly meetings with Shona's parents to keep them up to speed with how things are going at school and for them to share any concerns they might have. | Both parents and staff find this monthly meeting helpful as it means that Shona's parents are able to reinforce at home the kind of social messages that she is getting at school. The meetings are also a chance for the staff to celebrate Shona's achievements, which are easy to forget on a day-to-day basis. |
| Tracking behaviour outside school | This isn't felt to be necessary on a day-to-day basis but the regular meetings with her parents allow us to track any long-term changes that we might need to know about. | |
| Other | Shona has a lazy eye for which she has been recommended corrective surgery. She is anxious about this as she dislikes hospitals, almost to the point of phobia. She is, therefore, trying to convince everybody that she doesn't need her glasses (and therefore has no need for surgery) and will take them off and leave them lying around. This means that (a) she cannot see properly, which is dangerous in the playground and a nuisance in class, and (b) that her glasses, which are expensive because of the need for specialist lenses, are often damaged.<br><br>She needs to be reminded to keep them on and told – quite truthfully – that not wearing them means that she is more likely, not less, to need the surgery. | |

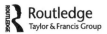

# Provision Record – Steven

| Name: Steven | National Curriculum year: 6 | School year beginning: 2011 |
|---|---|---|

| Situation | Provision | Reason for provision and potential outcome if it is not provided |
|---|---|---|
| **Arrival at school** | Though mum still brings Steven to school and takes him into the classroom, she is careful to leave quickly. | If mum hangs about Steven becomes more worked up because he's anticipating her leaving and can't cope with the prolonged anxiety that generates. |
| **Coming into classroom** | Once mum has left, Steven reads in the classroom or plays chess with a friend while the teacher is present but busy with her own tasks. | If Steven were left in the playground with the other children he would become anxious because he finds the noise and unpredictability of the other children distressing. He is also acutely aware of not being able to join in with playground activities as easily as the others do. |
| **Seating arrangements** | Steven sits at the back and to one side of the room with easy access to a spare table where he can work by himself if needed. | If Steven sits here, people don't have to be continually walking past him.<br><br>Although he doesn't need a work station, Steven does sometimes need to be able to work quietly by himself away from the distraction of other children. |
| **Toileting arrangements** | It has only recently come to light that Steven has never been to the toilet in school. (He never complained and it was only a chance comment from his mother that alerted us to this.) He is offered time during the lesson to go to the disabled toilet where it is quiet, because he does not like to think of people walking past outside and hearing him. It has taken him some time to get used to this but it is now working well. | Steven finds it uncomfortable and embarrassing to use the toilet when other people are nearby as he feels that they might hear or see him.<br><br>Obviously, there are medical issues that arise as a result of not going to the toilet and of not drinking enough during the school day. |

| Situation | Provision | Reason for provision and potential outcome if it is not provided |
|---|---|---|
| **Assembly** | Steven sits with his class at the end of a row next to somebody he gets on well with.<br><br>If the noise becomes too loud, he covers his ears and puts his chin down, so his TA watches for these signs. | If Steven had to sit in the middle of a row, he would find the noise and bustle (and the knowledge that he couldn't get away easily) difficult and stressful.<br><br>If he was not removed when the noise level got too high he would become anxious and wound up and this would lead to difficulties for Steven in attending to the following lesson. |
| **TA assistance** | There is a class TA who helps Steven as and when necessary, though the emphasis is on increasing his independence.<br><br>She will become involved if he is losing focus or getting stressed but is very aware of the need not to de-skill Steven or 'smother' him. | If Steven were unchecked and lost focus he would fall behind in his work. Through no fault of his own, Steven is easily distracted both by his own thoughts and by outside stimuli and, if he were not 'brought back', he would quickly lose the thread of his task and become anxious about not being able to complete it on time. |
| **Carpet time** | Not done in Year 5 in this school as sitting cross-legged on the ground is felt not to aid learning. | |
| **Sensory issues** | | |
| **Sound** | (See section on Assembly for effects on Steven of ambient noise.) | |
| **Taste and eating** | Because Steven has to have all foodstuffs separated on his plate at home, at school he eats a packed lunch in order to avoid this conflict. He does not like to be watched as he eats, so he eats in the classroom with the teacher working quietly. He also finds the sight of other people eating unpleasant. | If he were not allowed to eat by himself, Steven would not eat at all at school with obvious consequences for his blood sugar levels! |

| Situation | Provision | Reason for provision and potential outcome if it is not provided |
|---|---|---|
| Touch | If somebody accidentally knocks into him as he is walking to and fro in the corridor he misinterprets this as a deliberate act and assumes that whoever has bumped into him hates him. This requires the class TA to monitor what is happening and negotiate any misunderstandings.<br><br>He also dislikes tight or uncomfortable clothes and wears black jogging bottoms with elasticated waists instead of normal uniform trousers. His shoes are often undone as he does not like them to be tightly done up. | *[Authors' comments: Most people with an ASD will misinterpret non-intentional acts as having an intention. Comic strip conversations® can be useful in explaining the other child's point of view.]*<br><br>If he is uncomfortable Steven cannot concentrate and his work and behaviour suffer. This is not obvious in the classroom as Steven doesn't pull at his clothes or fidget, so we are reliant on advice and information from his parents on this subject. Discomfort due to clothing is very common for a child with an ASD. |
| Vision | N/A | |
| Smell | N/A | |
| Pairing | Steven can work with some children in the class but not others. The teacher will pair him with another child with whom he can work without becoming anxious or frustrated. | He would become anxious and frustrated if not paired appropriately. However, it is important that the other child is happy with this arrangement and, if not, the TA will act as Steven's partner.<br><br>If Steven were asked to work with someone less academically able he would become frustrated and might be 'rude' (unintentionally) to the other child. |
| Time awareness | Up until this year, Steven could read an analogue watch but, once he was taught digital time, his understanding of analogue seemed to vanish.<br><br>We have installed a digital clock in the class as well as an analogue one. | If we had just an analogue clock Steven would be unable to manage his work in terms of time. |

| Situation | Provision | Reason for provision and potential outcome if it is not provided |
|---|---|---|
| Specialist input | Steven is academically gifted and to extend his interest in philosophy and mathematics an ex-grammar school teacher visits twice a week to talk to Steven, once on his own and once as part of a small group.<br><br>A secondary school has been approached and Steven will be joining their science club once a week after school. | Steven looks forward to these sessions and if he did not have them in prospect he might become frustrated and bored with the curriculum. |
| Small group | As long as care is taken not to include children of a much lower ability in the same group, Steven is happy to work in a group. | If Steven works with children who are slower to catch on to what is required, he can be unintentionally rude and intolerant. (See section on Pairing.) |
| 1:1 work | As Steven is very capable academically, he does sometimes need extension work 'on the fly' from the class teacher, who can talk to him about issues arising from the subject under consideration. She might also allow Steven access to the class PC to answer questions that she does not have time for or know the answer to! | This keeps Steven interested and focused. Without this we feel he would become disengaged or actively frustrated.<br><br>It also helps in our goal of making Steven more independent if he can use the internet to research things for himself. He now needs encouragement (and some structural help) to make notes on this research so that he can record it. |
| Break | Steven's stress levels are monitored, and if he is having a particularly tense day he will be allowed to come in and read in the classroom.<br><br>However, most of the time, he is capable of joining in, at least at some level, with what is going on. | If he is unable to join in, Steven feels he is a failure and very quickly becomes depressed, with obvious consequences for his self-esteem. This means that he sometimes needs a little guidance from whoever is on duty. |

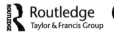

| Situation | Provision | Reason for provision and potential outcome if it is not provided |
|---|---|---|
| 'Who do I go to?' | In Steven's case this is not so much 'who' as 'where'. Steven has a very good relationship with his class teacher, who can arrange for him to leave the class for short breaks to sit in a quiet area, or engage the help of the SENCO as needed. | If not allowed to leave the class, he would become stressed and overwrought. Steven does not often take advantage of this facility but if he did not know that he could leave the class he would become far more anxious. |
| Lunchtime | After it was noticed that less effort was needed to get Steven to school on a Thursday, which was his library duty day, it was decided to allow him to do library duty at lunchtime every day apart from Friday when he plays board games with a carefully selected group of friends.<br><br>(See also section on Taste and eating.) | Steven finds an hour in the playground uncomfortable and he enjoys school far more knowing that he won't have to endure it. Library duty gives him a focus for interacting with the other children and means that he doesn't have to stress out about how to make social advances. |
| Motor difficulties, eg handwriting | Steven finds handwriting uncomfortable and is allowed to produce longer pieces of work on his laptop. However, so that he doesn't lose the skill of handwriting he is encouraged to do shorter items of work by hand.<br><br>He is being encouraged to learn to touch-type at home. | Steven would produce far less work than he is capable of if he wasn't allowed to use his laptop.<br><br>This is also a strategy that will be a useful life skill both in education and, subsequently, in work. |
| General organisational help | Steven is very organised, to the point where he likes things arranged neatly on his desk and has a very tidy drawer. He has no problems in organising his work. | |

| Situation | Provision | Reason for provision and potential outcome if it is not provided |
|---|---|---|
| **PE and swimming** | In Year 4 Steven was very loath to participate in any sorts of games; even when mum escorted him to swimming he was still unable to go into the pool. However, on entering Year 5 he almost naturally joined in with class sports and has done ever since. Swimming has not yet taken place but it is assumed that he will do this too. | *[Authors' comments: Always expect the unexpected!!*<br>*Always ensure that your support strategies do not prevent sudden changes of heart. Never say 'he never does that!'*<br>*And always give a child the opportunity to try something they have always backed away from before. A new term, a new school year or the arrival of a new teacher are all good times to try this.]* |
| **School trips** | Steven was unable to go on the four-day residential trip because he rarely sleeps more than three or four hours at night. Child and Adolescent Mental Health Services (CAMHS) have been consulted about this and the family are awaiting an appointment.<br><br>He is able to go on day trips without any difficulties, though the group he is in needs to be carefully selected and put under the class teacher's control. | If Steven's group were given to a parent helper, it's unlikely that Steven's particular needs would be understood and catered for. |
| **Variations, eg art week, book week** | Steven does not particularly like variations in the school routine. He finds sports day especially distressing as it is loud, different and competitive, He therefore doesn't come in on sports day because it offers him nothing and causes distress. Mum took him on a trip to a castle, which was beautifully quiet as it was during term time. | We think it's an example of not putting a square peg in a round hole! |

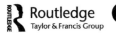

| Situation | Provision | Reason for provision and potential outcome if it is not provided |
|---|---|---|
| **Supply teachers** | Steven has no difficulties accepting a supply teacher, though the TA would monitor his reactions carefully. | |
| **Child's area of special interest** | See section on 1:1 work, which details provision for his special interest in philosophy. | |
| **Coping with inappropriate behaviour** | Steven displays no inappropriate or challenging behaviour at school, though it is reported that he does at home.<br><br>*[Authors' comment: This is very typical of ASD children; see 'A few helpful hints'.]* | It is only in talking to Steven's parents and hearing how Steven is when he gets home that we have realised just how stressful the school day is for him. This makes our stress-relieving strategies all the more important. |
| **Coping with meltdown** | Steven does not have meltdowns at school. | |
| **Homework** | Steven will do homework under duress, though he does not like it. We are sensitive to this as we do not wish to make home life any more difficult. | |
| **Liaison with parents** | There is a daily contact book stressing the positive side of every day because when Steven gets home tired and frustrated from working hard all day, he tends to focus on the negative aspects of his day. Parents can reaffirm the positive at the end of the day.<br><br>If parents want to contact school they do so via email rather than the book because Steven will read any comments as negative. | If Steven's day has been 90 per cent positive and 10 per cent negative, his parents will hear all about the 10 per cent and the 90 per cent will be ignored. This means that his parents can't help Steven to a more realistic and positive view of school and of his own competence. This is why stressing the positive both at home and school is so vital.<br><br>*[Authors' comment: See 'A few helpful hints'.]* |

| Situation | Provision | Reason for provision and potential outcome if it is not provided |
|---|---|---|
| **Tracking behaviour outside school** | This is done via regular, often daily, liaison with Steven's mother. | |
| Other | | |

Routledge
Taylor & Francis Group

## Tension thermometer

### Using the tension thermometer

We all know that individuals on the spectrum typically experience high levels of anxiety. It is also true that, for most, the higher their anxiety level, the less able they are to express it. The tension thermometer helps the child tell the adults in their environment how they are feeling without the need to speak. It can be used proactively if the child is happy to share their feelings, or the LSA can use it to ask how the child is feeling by showing the thermometer and asking discreetly 'Where are you now?'

Nb: The tension thermometer is designed to be used with children who have been given some help to understand their own emotions and to connect their own response with what's going on around them. Children who have not been given the vocabulary to talk about their emotional and bodily feelings would probably struggle to find the thermometer useful as they would not know how to identify the feelings of 'calm', and increasing 'tension' in their own case.

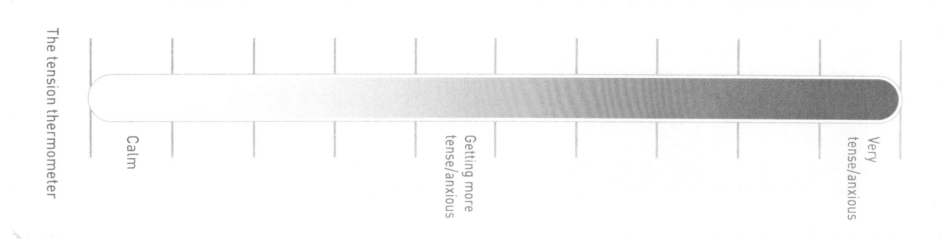

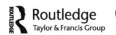

## Exit card

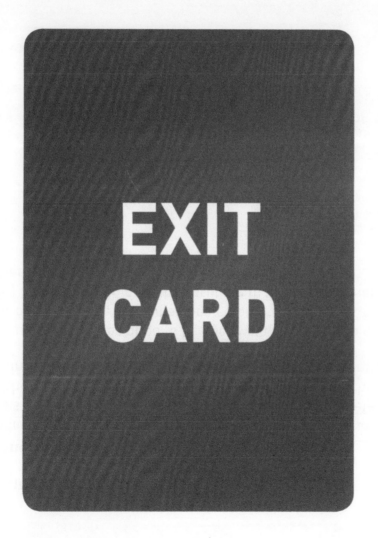

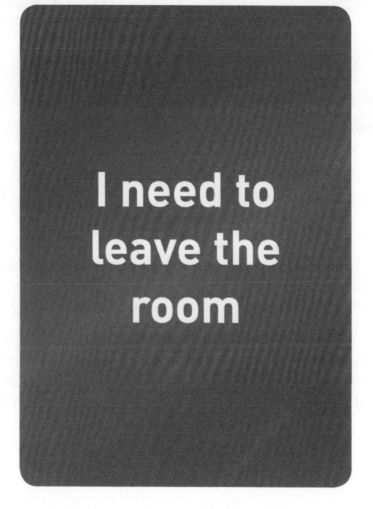

Ⓟ This page may be photocopied for instructional use only. *The Really Useful ASD Transition Pack* © Jan Newport and Alis Hawkins 2011

# Understanding measure

## Using the understanding measure

In our experience, some children on the autism spectrum find it difficult to ask for help and, as a consequence, they can flounder in lessons and get further and further behind, raising their anxiety levels and making it even more difficult for them to understand what's being said.

If the child with an ASD is able to be proactive, having the understanding measure somewhere easily accessible (pocket, pencil-case) enables them to signal to the learning support assistant that they need help, without having to verbalise the need. It can also be useful with children who lack the ability or confidence to be proactive – the LSA can point to the understanding measure and ask discreetly 'Where are you now?'

We have also seen the understanding measure used – very inclusively – as a whole-class strategy. Each child had an understanding measure taped to the desk in front of them and the class LSA wandered around the room monitoring each child's response to the teacher's input.

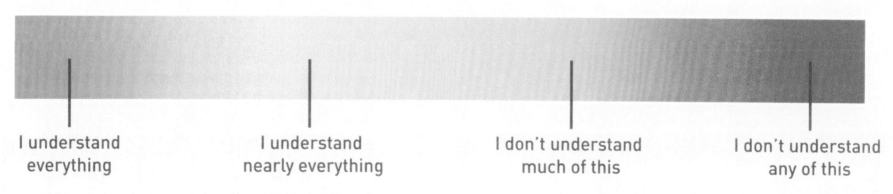

## Understanding measure

| I understand everything | I understand nearly everything | I don't understand much of this | I don't understand any of this |

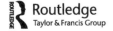

## Cue card showing how the child should set out each day's work in their book

Because of their high levels of anxiety and/or difficulties generalising skills from one situation to another, children on the spectrum will often ask, every day, how tasks should be done, even if this never varies significantly. This need to ask means that the child is dependent on adult input. If they have a cue card (shrunk down to a credit-card size and stowed in a pencil case or rendered in actual exercise-book size and stuck to the desk depending on the level of need) they can be more independent.

Initially, of course, there will be the learning period while the child is reminded to use the cue-card, but, over time, referring to it is likely to become automatic.

At the beginning of each lesson:

• Get your book and pencil case out

• Open your book to a new page

• Write down the date, title and learning objective like this:

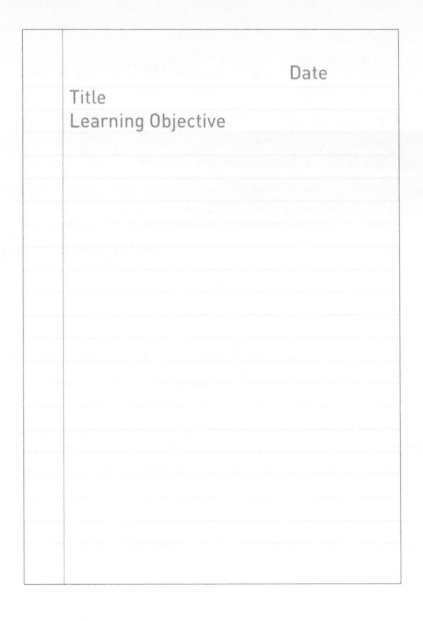

# Visual timetables

A visual timetable is simple to make using symbols or photographs and is a valuable tool in the classroom, especially for children who can't read yet or who find it difficult to relate to general class schedules on the board.

Visual timetables:

- **Give structure to the day** – children with an ASD sometimes find it difficult to remember the structure of the school day and may not realise that each day follows the same structure.

- **Promote independence** – so that children with an ASD will not have to keep asking 'what's next?' and can organise themselves (with help to begin with) and ensure that they have the right things for the next lesson.

- **Reduce anxiety** – not knowing where they are in the day or what is going to happen next can be very disorientating for children with an ASD and increase their anxiety unnecessarily.

- **Increase confidence** – children with an ASD do not have to depend on others and learn that they can organise their own equipment.

- **Build on the pupil's strength as a visual learner** – many children with an ASD have a preference for a visual learning style and can relate better to images and written words (which don't change and can be checked numerous times) than to spoken words (which disappear instantly and come back only if they keep asking the same question).

- **Build on the pupil's desire for routine, predictability and organisation** – many children with an ASD will be soothed by seeing that the structure of the day is predictable and can be checked and rechecked.

- **Give permanency** – because of common problems with time awareness and generalising things from one day to another, some children with an ASD can view each day as an event completely separate from all other days. Being able to see that each day in a week pans out in much the same way 'anchors' the child.

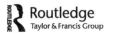

# Visual timetables

## Using the child's visual timetable

Obviously, there is no point simply having a visual timetable sitting on a child's desk or stuck on the wall – it has to be used in a way that is going to help the child. Each morning the class teacher or TA needs to go through the structure of the day with the child using the visual timetable, reminding them what each activity consists of, answering their questions, and reassuring them that help and support will be on hand for them all day. Being reassured of this – along with knowing what they are going to be doing during the day – will help to keep the child's anxieties to a minimum.

Below is the kind of visual timetable you might use with a foundation stage child. For children this young it is often more effective to use digital photographs of the child concerned doing these activities as, otherwise, they may not see the visual timetable as having anything to do with them. It's also good to name it for the younger child, for example 'Taylor's timetable'.

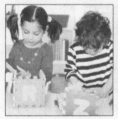 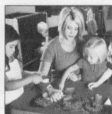 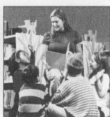 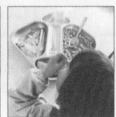 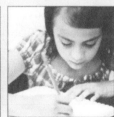 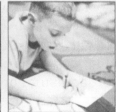 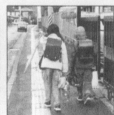 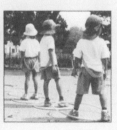

## Visual timetables

All the individual cards that make up the timetable should be attached to the base board using Velcro® or Blu Tack®. When each activity is finished the corresponding card should be put in a 'finished' box so that the child knows it is done with for the day.

A separate Velcro®-board which holds all the symbols can be very useful as then the child can be helped to construct their own timetable each morning.

Displayed below is what the timetable would look like at the end of the morning, just before lunch. The child has taken off all the 'completed' activity symbols and put them on the symbol board or the finished box, just leaving the afternoon's activities on the timetable. After lunch, the child will take off the lunch symbol, making it easy to see what will happen in the rest of the afternoon.

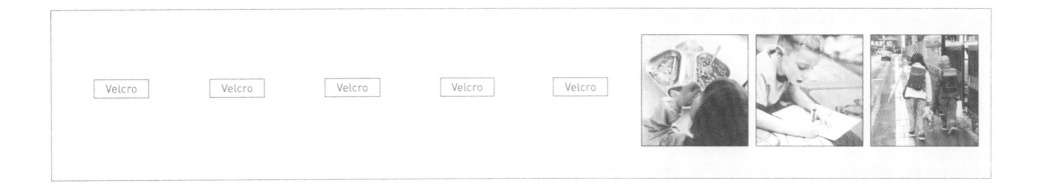

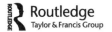

## More sophisticated visual timetables for older children

The visual timetable on page 103 represents the more sophisticated type that might be used with Key Stage 2 children or more able children in upper Key Stage 1.

Laminating the symbols will mean they last longer than a week!

It is important that you go through the timetable with the child before beginning to use it, to familiarise them with the symbols, especially if the child is not yet able to read or is progressing from a photograph-based timetable.

Older children can often cope better with a week at a time and, as they progress through Key Stage 2, it is useful for them to get used to seeing a week at a time because this prepares them for secondary school. However, it is important not to make too big a jump from a personalised, photographic, one-day-at-a-time timetable to a less personal, week-at-a-time one. A careful transition from one to the other may be needed, taking a one-day approach to begin with when the symbols are introduced.

To begin with, the child could continue to take the symbols off and put them in the finished box or on the symbol board but, as they progress towards Year 6, it is wise to help them scan through the symbols to find where they are in the day, if they are able to do this. This will also prepare the child for the use of timetables in secondary school.

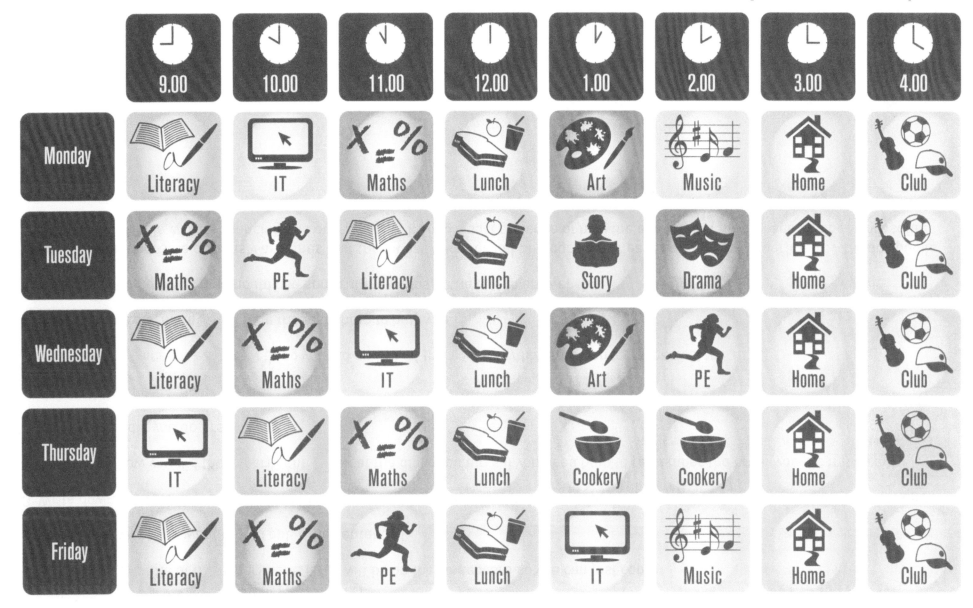

|  | 9.00 | 10.00 | 11.00 | 12.00 | 1.00 | 2.00 | 3.00 | 4.00 |
|---|---|---|---|---|---|---|---|---|
| Monday | Literacy | IT | Maths | Lunch | Art | Music | Home | Club |
| Tuesday | Maths | PE | Literacy | Lunch | Story | Drama | Home | Club |
| Wednesday | Literacy | Maths | IT | Lunch | Art | PE | Home | Club |
| Thursday | IT | Literacy | Maths | Lunch | Cookery | Cookery | Home | Club |
| Friday | Literacy | Maths | PE | Lunch | IT | Music | Home | Club |

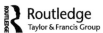

## Writing frame for science experiment

**1** Write down the title of the experiment. (This will be on the whiteboard so you can just copy it.)

**2** Write down what you want to find out. (One sentence.)

**3** Write down the title 'Equipment' and what equipment you used. (Do this as a list, putting each item of equipment on a different line.)

**4** Say exactly how you did the experiment. (Look at the digital pictures if you need help to remember the order you did things in.)

- What did you do first?

- What did you do next?

- Write a line for each new thing you did and say if there was anything you noticed at each step.

**5** How did the experiment end? (Use the last photo to help you.)

**6** What did you find out? (You should use some of the words in the title to answer this.)

**Note:** This writing frame obviously assumes that the TA has taken digital photographs of each stage of the experiment. As many pupils with an ASD struggle with sequencing and organisation, having visual evidence of how the experiment progressed can be very useful.

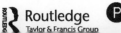

# Task breakdown sheet

| Subject: | Name: | Date: |
|---|---|---|

**TASK:** What do you have to do?

What materials/resources do you need to complete the task?

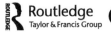

# Task breakdown sheet

**What do you have to do to complete the task correctly?**

**Time when task must be finished by**

1

2

3

Draw in clock face
or
write time
as appropriate.

This is the writing frame part.
Each element might have its own time frame.

4

5

6

7

Routledge
Taylor & Francis Group

# Task breakdown sheet

Some useful practical bits and pieces

Agreed reward for completing task satisfactorily:

This reward will be given if:

There will be no reward given if:

Routledge
Taylor & Francis Group

This page may be photocopied for instructional use only. *The Really Useful ASD Transition Pack* © Jan Newport and Alis Hawkins 2011

107

## 'I have had a fairly good day' sheet

The 'I have had a fairly good day' sheet is used occasionally for short perioas.

If a child is having fairly good days but going home and 'having a rant' as we are all prone to do, parents or teachers are able to use this sheet, firstly to put the 'bad stuff' in proportion and secondly to affirm good things that have happened in the day.

There is nothing wrong with 'having a rant'; it allows us to let off steam. However, a child with an ASD will often focus only on the bad and not remember the good, and if this is left unsupported it can lead to an unbalanced view of their day and possible school refusal.

Parents generally welcome the chance to discuss 'good things' with their child.

The form can be easily adapted to suit the individual child and your school.

The child is asked to reflect after each lesson and either a short sentence can be written, saying what happened and how the child felt, or 'smiley face' stickers can be used.

## 'I have had a fairly good day' sheet

- Lesson 1 ........................................................................

- Lesson 2 ........................................................................

- Lesson 3 ........................................................................

- LUNCH 4 ........................................................................

- Lesson 5 ........................................................................

- Lesson 6 ........................................................................


There was a bit of my day I did not like .........................

........................................................................

There was a bit of my day I really liked .........................

........................................................................

Colour in the proportion that you did not like and see how much of the day was OK

| | | | | | | | | | |
|---|---|---|---|---|---|---|---|---|---|
| | | | | | | | | | |

Overall my day was OK. ☺

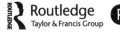

Although we have said that inflexibility is part and parcel of ASD, it may help you to consider the following:

## Varying the routine in your classroom

Although some children with an ASD need as little change as possible, to prevent them becoming too 'set in their ways' and resistant to change, as their anxiety reduces, some small, planned changes can help them to be more flexible and accepting of variations to routine.

If you use a central pot of pencils, instead of each child having their own pencils in their tray, swap the colours around the different tables regularly – red ones on the table one day or one week, green ones the next. Make a game of it – ask the children what colour pot of pencils was on their table yesterday and see if they can remember. (The child with an ASD probably will remember and you can celebrate their ability to notice things!)

You could write the date on the board in green and surround it with a square one day, in blue surrounded by a circle the next, and see if the children can tell you what yesterday's shape was.

If the child with an ASD sits on a table with other children, get everybody to swap places and see if the children can remember who was sitting in their seat before. You will be able to think of other things appropriate for your particular child with an ASD. But remember, do this only when the child seems relaxed and happy in the classroom.

# Be prepared for unexpected changes

Always keep an open mind to the possibility that the child may suddenly be able to do something they have always resisted before. Be careful not to put up barriers through your own attitude, even if you think you are being kind to the child. ASD is a developmental disorder and a child may suddenly mature in one particular area, making it possible for them to do things they could not previously do.

For instance, a child who has always been unable to join in with swimming may suddenly decide they can do it in Year 4.

It is important always to give children the opportunity to do things even if they have never shown any ability to do them before. Never say, 'He doesn't do that'.

So that you don't make the child self-conscious, it is probably better not to draw attention to this sort of sudden change, even if your immediate impulse is to congratulate the child and point out that they have done something for the first time. It is probably best to stick to a simple 'Well done!' This probably sounds counter-intuitive but children with an ASD often hate having attention drawn to themselves and, if they feel that they are going to be singled out for attention, they may feel too self-conscious ever to attempt to do something new again.

# Glossary

**CAMHS:** Child and Adolescent Mental Health Services.

**Comic Strip Conversation®:** a technique developed by Carol Gray whereby pictures of stick men, incorporating speech bubbles (what people said) and thought bubbles (what their thoughts and motivations were) are used to help children on the autism spectrum understand social interactions.

**Communicate: SymWriter®:** a simple word processor that uses symbols.

**Fizzy:** a programme designed by physiotherapists to be delivered by school staff to aid co-ordination, sequencing, balance etc.

**Joint attention:** the process in which one person draws the attention of another to an object by a non-verbal behaviour like eye-gaze, nodding or pointing. For example, if a baby wants to tell his father he has seen an aeroplane in the sky, he might make eye contact with his father, then look at the plane and look back to his father to make sure that he has 'shared' attention to the same object. In any episode of joint attention there is always a person who initiates the exchange, another who is invited to share attention and an object to be attended to. Joint attention is a precursor to 'theory of mind' (see below).

**Meltdown:** an episode of unwanted behaviour arising from the child with an ASD being overloaded with information, demands or anxiety. Meltdowns can result in externalising behaviour – shouting, screaming, throwing things, self-injurious behaviours, injuring others; or internalising behaviour – becoming intensely withdrawn and non-verbal, often seeking sanctuary (curling up (going foetal) under a desk, running out of the school) and being unresponsive to questions or attempts by those around the child to engage with them.

**Mind Maps®:** a visual technique for thinking, organising and remembering information developed by Tony Buzan.

**SENCO:** special educational needs co-ordinator (sometimes AENCO: additional educational needs co-ordinator).

**Social Stories™:** a technique developed by Carol Gray to help children with learning difficulties to understand and respond more acceptably to social situations.

**TA:** teaching assistant.

**Theory of mind:** the ability to attribute mental states – that is emotions, beliefs, imaginative states, knowledge – to oneself and other people. It includes the ability to understand that other people have their own thoughts, beliefs and emotions which are separate and different from one's own. Seen in typically-developing children by 2-3 years of age. Commonly significantly delayed in those with an ASD.

**Writing frames:** a technique which gives the child an outline to structure their writing so that they can concentrate on the *content* of what they are writing rather than struggling with the *form* they need to use.

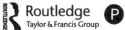

# Suggested reading list

**Attwood T** (1998) *Asperger's Syndrome: A Guide for Parents and Professionals*, Jessica Kingsley Publishers, London.

**Cumine V, Dunlop J & Stevenson G** (1998) *Asperger Syndrome: A Practical Guide for Teachers*, David Fulton Publishers, London.

**Grandin T** (1995) *Thinking in Pictures: And Other Reports From my Life with Autism*, Doubleday, New York.

**Jackson L** (2002) *Freaks, Geeks and Asperger Syndrome: A User Guide to Adolescence*, Jessica Kingsley Publishers, London.

**Myles B S & Southwick J** (2005) *Asperger's Syndrome and Difficult Moments: Practical Solutions for Tantrums, Rage and Meltdowns*, Autism Asperger Publishing, Shawnee Mission, KS, USA.

**Sainsbury C** (2009) *The Martian in the Playground: Understanding the Schoolchild with Asperger's Syndrome*, Sage Publications, London.

**Seach D, Lloyd M & Preston M** (2003) *Supporting Children with Autism in Mainstream Schools*, Questions Publishing Company, London.

For Product Safety Concerns and Information please contact our EU representative GPSR@taylorandfrancis.com Taylor & Francis Verlag GmbH, Kaufingerstraße 24, 80331 München, Germany

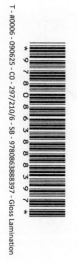

T - #0006 - 090625 - C0 - 297/210/6 - SB - 9780863888397 - Gloss Lamination